Natural Healing for Men

From the heart to the prostate, from ulcers to the common cold, herbs have an important role to play in supporting men's health. They tone and strengthen all systems of the body, restore mental, emotional and physical balance and enhance immunity. Whether it's ginseng for stamina, arnica for injuries, kava kava for stress or saw palmetto for the prostate, herbs often work as well as or even better (and certainly less expensively) than prescription drugs—and without their unpleasant and sometimes dangerous side effects. Choose the herbs that are right for you with the help of this invaluable guide.

About the Author

CJ Puotinen has studied with some of America's leading herbalists and is a member of the Herb Research Foundation, the American Herb Association, the International Herb Association and the Northeast Herbal Association. In addition to magazine and journal articles on health and medicinal herbs, she is the author of *Herbal Teas, Nature's Antiseptics: Tea Tree Oil and Grapefruit Seed Extract, Herbs to Improve Digestion* and *Herbs to Help You Breathe Freely,* all published by Keats Publishing, Inc.

A KEATS GOOD HERB GUIDE

MEDICINE FOR THE 21ST CENTURY

HERBS FOR MEN'S HEALTH

CJ Puotinen

Keats Publishing, Inc. New Canaan, Connecticut

Herbs for Men's Health is intended solely for informational and educational purposes, and not as medical advice. Please consult a medical or health professional if you have questions about your health.

HERBS FOR MEN'S HEALTH

Library of Congress Cataloging-in-Publication Data

Puotinen, CJ
Herbs for men's better health / CJ Puotinen.
p. cm.—(A Keats good herb guide)
Includes bibliographical references and index.
ISBN 0-87983-782-9
1. Herbs—Therapeutic use. 2. Men—Health and hygiene.
I. Title II. Series.
RM666.H33P86 1997
615'.321'081—dc21 96-36934
CIP

Printed in the United States of America

Published by Keats Publishing, Inc.
27 Pine Street (Box 876)
New Canaan, Connecticut 06840-0876

98 97 96 6 5 4 3 2 1

Contents

For Joel,
the man in my life

Introduction

Whether it's ginseng for stamina and virility, arnica for sports injuries, kava kava for stress, gotu kola for improved memory, saw palmetto for the prostate, tea tree oil for athlete's foot or cayenne pepper for the heart, certain herbs have a special affinity for the male system.

What few Americans realize is that many herbs work as well as or better than prescription drugs or surgery, claims repeatedly proven by medical researchers in the U.S. and around the world. However, that's changing as more physicians treat medical problems with diet, herbs and nutritional supplements, a strategy that corrects the underlying cause of illness and avoids the adverse side effects of more orthodox therapies.

One of the most common medical procedures today is bypass surgery. Typically, a middle-aged man is told, "You are a walking time bomb. Unless we operate immediately, you're going to die."

Is that true? According to Julian Whitaker, M.D., the answer is almost always no. His advice: Never agree to immediate surgery. Instead, get a second opinion, and before doing that, consider the evidence.

In 1977, results of an ambitious Veterans Administration Cooperative Study that tested bypass surgery were published. The scientifically controlled trial of 596 patients, all with the same degree of blocked arteries, concluded that surgery was no better than conventional medications at preventing heart attacks or saving lives. The patients were randomly assigned to receive either medical therapy or bypass surgery, and the death rate in both groups was identical.

The study was not well-received by surgeons, who demanded a new trial. The government then spent 100 million dollars on the Coronary Artery Surgical Study, or CASS. This time 780 patients with severely blocked arteries were divided into two groups, one of which received surgery, the other conventional medical therapy. The results, published in 1983, showed that for the average patient, the risk of dying from bypass surgery is three to five times greater than the risk of dying from heart disease. In an editorial accompanying the CASS study, Eugene Braunwald, M.D., then chief of cardiology at Harvard Medical School, predicted that the use of bypass surgery would decrease because of its ineffectiveness.

Obviously, that didn't happen. Why are so many men receiving bypass operations? As Dr. Whitaker explains,

> If the profession followed the recommendations of its own scientific studies, the heart surgery industry would collapse overnight. In order for that industry to survive and flourish, it must perform large numbers of totally unnecessary procedures. And since that industry churns out about 1,000 newly minted heart surgeons each year, all eager to ply their craft "helping folks" with this terrible disease, the heart patient with just a little heart disease swims with sharks in a feeding frenzy. Friends, this is not a scientific debate among hard-working, concerned physicians doing their best to help their patients. This is fraud on a monstrous scale.

For most of the 20th century, physicians insisted that there is no link between diet and heart disease, that heart disease is irreversible and incurable and that the only appropriate treatments are symptom-suppressing drugs and surgery.

Then Nathan Pritikin cured his own heart disease with a low-fat diet, and his health centers trained thousands of people to do the same. Still, physicians were skeptical. It wasn't until Dean Ornish conducted a clinical trial at the University of California that the medical establishment realized that heart disease can be not only stopped but reversed and cured by changes in diet and lifestyle.

Then there's the prostate industry.

At birth, a boy's prostate gland is the size of a grain of wheat. It grows through adolescence until reaching the size of a chestnut, at which point growth stops. However, in middle age, the prostate again expands. Although medical researchers assume the renewed growth has something to do with hormone production, no one has been able to explain how or why it happens.

The result, called benign prostatic hypertrophy, or BPH, causes symptoms that range from mildly irritating to life-threatening. Typically, a man begins to notice that he's spending more time in the bathroom. The need to urinate may be strong and urgent, especially at night, but the resulting stream is scanty and the effort painful. This is because the swollen prostate exerts pressure that produces a feeling of fullness and interferes with urine flow.

Enter Proscar, the most popular drug treatment for enlarged prostates. Proscar (finasteride) must be taken for three to six months before symptoms improve, and they do so in only a small minority of patients. In fact, in August 1996, *The New England Journal of Medicine* announced that when tested on over 1,200 men at 31 Veterans Administration medical centers, Proscar gave "no greater relief than the placebo." Proscar does shrink the prostate gland, but as Dr. Herbert Lepor, chairman of urology at New York University Medical Center, explained,

''This study not only confirms that there is no need to do that, but also that shrinking the gland has no significant effect on symptom relief.'' Proscar's side effects are better documented. In an earlier trial of 543 patients, seven had to stop treatment because of adverse reactions. Side effects include impotence, decreased libido, breast tenderness and enlargement, a skin rash and swollen lips. In addition, Proscar's greatest dangers are to its users' wives, unborn children and young boys. Pregnant women should never touch Proscar or have unprotected sex with a man who is taking it because his semen could damage a male fetus, and the drug must be kept away from children of all ages.

Are there alternatives to prescription drugs? See pages 51–56 for herbal therapies that outperform Proscar and bring well-documented relief from BPH.

In prostate circles, the big money lies in cancer screening and treatment, often immediate surgery, radiation and/or chemotherapy. Here the side effects are more dramatic, for they include severe pain, lengthy disability, incontinence, impotence and immune system disruption. Does early intervention save lives or improve the quality of life? No evidence supports this approach. For decades, Swedish men with prostate cancer have been treated with ''watchful waiting'' until the cancer emerges from the capsule of the prostate and causes symptoms, which statistics show seldom happens. There is no difference in survival rates: a man with untreated prostate cancer is as likely to die of heart disease or other causes 10 to 20 years after diagnosis as he is to die of cancer. The most famous American study verifying the Swedish approach is the SEER program (Surveillance, Epidemiology and End Results) conducted by the Center for Evaluative Clinical Sciences in Hanover, N.H. The study found that while prostate cancer increased only modestly in America during the 1980s, prostate surgery increased at the rate of 35 percent per year and even more in some parts of the country. While the surgeries were profitable to hospitals and physicians, they did not save lives. In 1994, the *New England Journal of Medicine* endorsed ''watchful waiting'' rather than aggressive intervention for nearly all prostate cancers detected in older men.

Heart disease and swollen prostates are only two of the medical conditions common to American men. They and a host of other ailments can be improved, treated, reversed and in some cases cured by methods other than drugs and surgery—and often the most successful, well documented, effective treatments involve medicinal herbs.

Herbal medicine has such a long history, its origins are lost in the mists of time. Like our fellow animals, people have been treating themselves with plants for millennia. Most of the prescription drugs sold today are derived from plants, and pharmaceutical companies still send botanists to distant rain forests in the search for cures.

There are two approaches to using plant-based medicines. One is to isolate the plant's active ingredient and synthesize it in order to create a patented drug. The other is to use the plant itself, with all of its constituents. The first approach is refined, the second, crude. Crude plant extracts and whole leaf teas provide not only the plant's active ingredients, but dozens of interacting chemicals that may have a profound effect on the person taking them. In many cases, the same plant contains both a toxic component and its antidote.

For example, sassafras contains safrole, a substance that the FDA tested in large quantities on rats in the 1950s. When the rats developed liver cancer, sassafras was blamed. The same compound, safrole, is found in nutmeg, black pepper and mace, but these seasonings were never implicated. Because safrole is not soluble in water, someone drinking sassafras tea will ingest very little of it, and no case of liver damage from sassafras tea has ever been reported. In fact, the southeastern U.S., where most sassafras tea is consumed, has a lower liver cancer rate than other parts of the country. There are so many chemical compounds in sassafras and their interactions are so complicated that no one understands how they work. However, botanical researchers suggest that sassafras contains ingredients that prevent safrole from harming the liver and which may, in fact, strengthen that organ. All plants contain a complicated matrix of chemical compounds and, to date, no synthetic product, whether an essential oil, flavoring agent or drug, has ever duplicated Mother Nature.

The Safety of Herbs

To say that herbal medicine is controversial is to make an understatement. Warnings about their use abound. In 1983, *FDA Consumer,* a U.S. Department of Health and Human Services magazine, published a lengthy article titled, "Herbs Are Often More Toxic Than Magical."

The article offered six "cautions" to anyone considering taking an herb for medicinal use. These cautions are widely quoted and reflect the FDA's concerns about the safety and appropriateness of herbal therapies.

Caution One: Some herbs contain the wrong kind of magic; some are potent poisons, like hemlock, curare and deadly nightshade. That's true, and no one recommends using these plants as teas. Mislabeled herbs and toxic contaminants are certainly possible, but reputable herb companies, especially those that specialize in wildcrafted and organically grown plants, have an excellent safety record.

Caution Two: We don't know enough about herbal teas to conclude that they are safe. "Manufacturers of herbal teas have not submitted their products to FDA or made the required animal studies for a determination of safety," says the article. One reason the FDA knows so little about herb safety is that it does not recognize research conducted in foreign countries, such as Germany, Austria, England and Japan, and critics claim that it often ignores the evidence supplied by American universities and researchers.

Because herbs cannot be patented, there is no economic

incentive for their testing in the United States, where proving the effectiveness and safety of a drug to the FDA's satisfaction can take 10 or more years and cost 100 million dollars.

Caution Three: Doctoring yourself with herbs can be very dangerous. "Given the availability of modern medicines with proven effectiveness and safety when used as directed," warns the FDA, "treating ailments with herbs is both unnecessary and risky."

If orthodox therapies worked, would people of all socioeconomic and educational backgrounds invest billions of dollars every year in alternatives? Orthodox medicine's failure to cure chronic illnesses like arthritis, asthma, heart disease, diverticulitis and prostatitis results from its failure to address the cause of disease.

A large percentage of FDA-approved drugs are withdrawn from the market within a few years of their release because of adverse side effects that were not discovered or not reported during testing, side effects that are often fatal or debilitating. Few people know that at least half of the most widely used allopathic therapies are themselves unproven, including chemotherapy for cancer, heart bypass surgery, hysterectomies, the ultrasound screening of unborn babies, surgery for back pain, radical mastectomy to cure breast cancer, drugs to lower blood pressure or cholesterol, radiation or surgery for prostate tumors, hormone replacement therapy and balloon angioplasty to unblock heart arteries. Critics like Julian Whitaker and award-winning medical journalist Lynne McTaggart cite research published in highly regarded medical journals showing that these therapies have never been proven effective, but because they are so profitable to hospitals, physicians and drug companies, they remain widely prescribed.

It is possible to create problems if you self-treat with the wrong medicinal plants, but in general, the risks of self-treatment are far less than those experienced by most hospital patients, whose infections and misfortunes have made iatrogenic (physician-caused) illness a widespread phenomenon. Deaths from herbal medications are so rare, they make headlines. Deaths from prescription drug overdoses, prescription drug side effects, over-the-counter medications and medical staff errors are so common that they go unnoticed.

Caution Four: Moderation in all things. The excessive consumption of any food or plant can be harmful. No argument here; it's common sense advice, which applies as much to the overconsumption of tobacco, alcohol and antibiotics as it does to the use of herbs.

Caution Five: Not all men are created equal, nor women either. This caution refers to individual reactions, which vary from person to person.

Most of the herbs described here are regarded as safe even in large doses (those that are not are clearly labeled), but individual reactions vary. Always start with a small amount of an herb you are taking for the first time and pay close attention to your body's response. If you develop any adverse symptom, such as a rash, nausea, rapid heart rate, dizziness, headache, itching or difficulty in breathing, trust your experience and discontinue its use. Even herbs generally recognized as safe may cause an allergic reaction in some people, and any herb taken in excess may be harmful.

Caution Six: Remember the old, bold mushroom hunter. There are old mushroom hunters and bold mushroom hunters, but there are no old, bold mushroom hunters. The same is true for anyone who collects plants in the wild without exercising caution. Reliable sources and careful identification are essential.

The Herb Research Foundation (see Resources) gathers scientific data pertaining to herb safety from around the world and publishes inexpensive reports and tables comparing the carcinogenic potential of common herbs and foods. If you're concerned about the safety and scientific testing of any medicinal herb, send a self-addressed stamped envelope to the Herb Research Foundation requesting information.

In conclusion, common sense and education are your best guides to herb use. Don't use an herb without learning about it first. Mislabeled herbs are rare, but a company that grows its own herbs and tests what it buys insures product safety. The safest herbs may be those you grow yourself using organic methods or those you purchase from reputable sources. Unfortunately, nearly all herbs imported into the United States are fumigated or otherwise treated with chemicals, a consideration for anyone using herbs medicinally. No discussion of herb safety would be complete without a mention of this concern. Whenever possible, buy herbs from organic or wildcrafted U.S. sources or grow them yourself.

How to Use Herbs

Herbs can be eaten raw, added to foods, brewed as teas, taken in capsules or tablets, applied externally, made into tinctures or liquid extracts and distilled into highly concentrated essential oils.

To judge the quality of a dried herb, such as the contents of an herbal tea bag or box of loose tea, spread the tea on a flat surface and inspect it. Can you recognize the plant? If it looks, smells and tastes like chamomile, with bright yellow blossoms that have a pronounced apple fragrance, you probably have a high quality chamomile. If it's indistinguishable from straw or sawdust, you don't.

Whole leaves and blossoms hold their fragrance, color and medicinal properties longer than cut or chopped herbs, which in turn remain active longer than powdered herbs.

How long can herbs be stored before use? Herbs in well-sealed amber glass jars that are protected from heat and light can be potent for years, while finely ground or powdered herbs stored in unsealed containers near heat, light and humidity may lose their effectiveness in weeks.

Learn to trust your nose, eyes and taste buds. Compare brands. Experiment. Discard any dried herbs that seem tired or taste like cardboard and any tinctures that are colorless, flavorless and odorless. Look for deep color, pungent fragrances, firm texture and sharp tastes, all of which indicate careful harvesting, low temperature drying and proper storage.

TEAS. To prepare an **infusion**, the preferred method for brewing most teas composed of leaves and blossoms, pour 1 cup (8 ounces) boiling water over 1 tsp. dried tea in a covered container. Let stand 10 minutes, strain and serve. These proportions of water and herbs brew a beverage strength tea. For a medicinal tea, brewed to treat a specific condition, use 2 to 3 tsp. (1 Tbsp.) dried herb per 1 cup of water and let the infusion stand ½ hour to several hours or overnight. For convenience, brew 2 cups (1 pint) or 4 cups (1 quart) at a time.

To prepare a **decoction**, the preferred method for brewing most teas composed of barks and roots, use the same proportions of tea and water but place them in a covered pan, bring to a boil and simmer over low heat for 10 to 15 minutes; let stand an additional 5 minutes, strain and serve.

Teas can be sweetened with sugar or honey, although for medicinal purposes, most herbalists recommend unsweetened tea. Preferred sweeteners include stevia, which is sold as a liquid concentrate or dried herb, and fruit juice or juice concentrates.

TINCTURES are liquid extracts made by soaking fresh or dried herbs in grain alcohol such as rum or vodka, vegetable glycerine or a combination of both. Tinctures have a long shelf life and are concentrated, especially if made with a sufficient quantity of plant material and aged for several weeks before straining.

Despite their concentration, tinctures aren't as strong as their labels suggest. According to Rosemary Gladstar, who pioneered popular herbology in the 1960s and is one of America's foremost herbalists, the miniscule doses on most tincture labels date back to the early days of commercial tincture making when the only comparable products were homeopathic. In homeopathy, doses are measured by the drop. For lack of a better system of dosages, herbalists used similar measurements. In most cases, Gladstar asserts, when a tincture bottle recommends 15 to 20 drops, you'd do better to take half a teaspoon or even a tablespoon, depending on the herbs involved and the condition you're treating. Keep this in mind if you ever find an herbal tincture ineffective. It may be that the herb is working fine, but the dosage isn't.

CAPSULES contain cut and sifted, chopped or powdered herbs. Because powdered herbs lose their potency when exposed to heat, light or humidity, they should be purchased from a reliable source and stored carefully. Kitchen cabinets near the stove are not a good place to store medicinal herbs, whether teas or capsules. For long-range storage, consider a cool, dark basement or even the refrigerator or freezer.

One way to insure quality capsules is to obtain high-grade dried herbs, grind them yourself in any coffee or spice grinder and fill your own. Two-part gelatin capsules (including vegetarian capsules) come in three sizes, as do hand-operated capping devices that make filling them easy work. Some herb companies will blend and grind herbs and place them in capsules for you, and health food stores carry an increasing variety of herbal capsules.

ESSENTIAL OILS, the basis of aromatherapy, are the most concentrated extracts available. Several pounds of plant material, usually leaves and blossoms, are needed to make an ounce of distilled essential oil. This explains why essential oils are so expensive and why aromatherapy books contain so many cautions about their use. A few drops go a long way. Most essential oils are far too concentrated to use full strength, especially on the skin, but one exception is tea tree oil, which is well-tolerated by most adults. Essential oils are used for fragrance, as in colognes and after-shave products; some are effective insect repellents; others are natural antidepressants or energy stimulating; and some, like tea tree oil, have a variety of therapeutic uses. See pages 73–78 for AROMATHERAPY information.

MASSAGE OILS are blends of "carrier oils," such as olive or almond oil, with a few drops of herbal essential oil or they are carrier oils in which fresh or dried herbs were infused or heated. They often contain relaxing or antispasmodic herbs and herbs that improve capillary circulation to speed the healing of sprains and bruises.

Herbs for Men

The following herbs are effective in treating the most common problems experienced by American men today. Except for arnica and tea tree oil, which should not be taken internally, they can be used separately or together in any of the forms described above.

Keep in mind that individual reactions vary, and anyone might have an allergic or unpleasant reaction to any plant, just as some people are allergic to strawberries and others to peanuts or shellfish. For best results, work with a physician, nutritionist or herbalist who has extensive experience with botanical medicines, study the recommended reading list, buy your herbs from reputable and reliable sources and use organically grown or wildcrafted herbs whenever possible.

Some of the following herbs are "specifics" or single-herb remedies for specific conditions. Saw palmetto berry, for example, is a specific for the prostate; hawthorn berry is a specific for the heart. These herbs can be used alone, in which case they are called "simples." However, most of the herbs listed here are used in blends; they are combined with herbs that have compatible or similar uses and with "catalyst" herbs, which have a stimulating effect, for improved performance. While you may not be interested in blending your own herbal teas, tinctures and capsules, you will find hundreds of combinations in your health food store and herbal product catalogs. To decipher their labels and determine which blend is most likely to treat your condition, refer to the following descriptions.

When studying labels, remember that in the U.S. the ingredient used in the largest amount must be listed first. A prostate blend containing saw palmetto berry, pygeum, goldenrod and cayenne pepper might contain equal parts of these four ingredients, but it is more likely to contain more saw palmetto berry and less cayenne pepper than anything else.

Stimulant or catalyst herbs, like cayenne, sarsaparilla, rosemary, prickly ash bark, ginger root, sage and astragalus, are often among the last herbs listed on a blend's label because they are used in small quantities. These herbs stimulate blood circulation and digestion to enhance the performance of the blend's other herbs, much the way that caffeine does when it is added to aspirin products.

ALCOHOL, NUTRITION AND HERBS FOR LIVER HEALTH

Heavy drinking, like cigarette smoking, does much to harm and little to help the body. Both activities are addictive and lead to nutritional imbalances that contribute to serious illnesses and symptoms such as impotence.

Alcoholics who have quit drinking usually avoid alcohol tinctures of medicinal herbs, but some companies make low-alcohol tinctures, substitute vegetable glycerine for alcohol or remove the alcohol before bottling. Pouring boiling water over an alcohol tincture will remove some though not all of its alcohol; this method is widely used to lower the alcohol content of medicinal tinctures.

Experiments with mice, and later with humans, showed a strong link between vitamin B deficiencies and alcohol cravings. A good multivitamin with additional B-complex supplementation (at least 50 mg each of vitamin B-6 and niacinamide) and a trace mineral supplement daily, plus 1 gram (1000 mg) of the amino acid glutamine taken 3 times daily on an empty stomach, will significantly reduce alcohol cravings and correct the nutritional deficiencies most common to alcoholics.

The herbs kudzu and milk thistle seed are important to heavy drinkers and those who have stopped drinking; the former helps reduce the craving for alcohol and the latter repairs liver damage.

Kudzu (*Pueraria lobata*)

In the early 1990s, the most disliked weed in the American South made headlines. Research published in the *Proceedings of the National Academy of Sciences* tested the vine's starchy root on golden hamsters, a species notorious for its capacity and craving for alcohol. An extract of kudzu dramatically reduced alcohol consumption in alcoholic hamsters. Kudzu tea has been used for centuries in China and Japan to treat alcoholism, a use that prompted this study because of its alleged effectiveness. Note that kudzu tea, made from the whole root, is different from kudzu starch sold in health food stores. The starch, used by Japanese cooks as a thickening agent much like cornstarch, is made by grinding kudzu roots in water, letting the starch settle out, pouring away the residue and repeating this process until a pure fine white powder results. In this processing, kudzu's water-soluble constituents are washed away.

In China, clinical studies conducted in the 1970s verified the effectiveness of crude kudzu root preparations in the treatment of high blood pressure, migraine headaches and aching shoulders and muscles. Kudzu's flavonoids, which are believed to be the plant's active medicinal ingredients, increase blood flow and relieve intestinal cramping by reducing the contraction of smooth muscle tissue. Chinese researchers have treated sudden deafness, which can be caused by impaired blood circulation, and circulatory problems with kudzu flavonoids.

To reduce cravings for alcohol and to reduce alcohol consumption, look for *pueraria* in health food stores or herb tea catalogs, where it is likely to be labeled by its Latin name, or look for imported *kakkon* (kudzu root tea), which may contain ginger, licorice and cinnamon as well. A few natural food stores and Chinese pharmacies carry kudzu root tablets and tinctures under the names *ge-gen* or *ko-ken*. Some kudzu products have English names like "Before and After," as in before and after partying, in which case follow package directions. If you're using dried *pueraria* or kudzu root, brew a decoction by simmering 1 tsp. dried herb per 1 cup of water for 10 to 15 minutes in a covered pan; let stand a few minutes, strain and serve. One cup of tea before cocktails should help reduce cravings; a cup after drinking may help reduce hangover symptoms.

If you live in the Southeast and have access to kudzu vines that grow far from busy highways and other sources of pollution, you can dig your own roots, scrub them off, chop them into small pieces and let them dry in a warm dry shady place with ample air circulation until they're completely dry. Store in tightly sealed glass jars or plastic bags away from heat and light.

Milk Thistle Seed (*Sylybum marianum*)

Environmental toxins, alcohol and a variety of other substances put daily stress on your liver, immune system, nervous system and emotions. Detoxification, regeneration and protection are the bywords of herbalists and nutritionally oriented physicians, who use plants to repair the damage. One of their favorite herbs is milk thistle seed, which is so effective it can regenerate almost any liver, even one damaged by poisonous mushrooms, hepatitis, drugs or cirrhosis.

The large gray seeds of the milk thistle enjoy an impressive reputation after nearly 50 years of European research, where pharmaceutical-grade milk thistle extracts are made for hypodermic injection as well as oral consumption. The seeds strengthen and tone the liver, are mucilaginous and soothing to the entire system and promote the flow of bile to improve digestion.

Animal and human tests of milk thistle seed indicate that even when taken in large doses, adverse side effects are extremely rare. The only adverse reaction has been a mild laxative effect in isolated cases.

In addition to stimulating liver regeneration in cases of mushroom poisoning, liver disease and alcohol abuse, milk thistle seed is one of the most powerful yet gentle herbs for detoxification. It protects against common airborne pollutants distributed by the smoke of burning wood, tobacco, coal, oil and many commercially prepared incense products. In addition, the seed protects against X-rays and the side effects of radiation therapy.

Milk thistle seed can be ground and added to food or brewed as a tea, but it is usually taken as a tincture (1/4 tsp. or more daily, as needed) or in capsule form (1 capsule 3 or 4 times daily). Like many herbs, milk thistle seed has a gradual influence and a course of treatment lasting at least three months is recommended before judging its effect.

HERBAL APHRODISIACS

Do herbal aphrodisiacs work? In some cases, yes. Yohimbe, damiana, ginseng, green oats and stinging nettle have received impressive testimonials from satisfied users.

The same herbs, however, have had no effect on some who tried them. One complication may be prescription drugs, for antihistamines, antidepressants, antibiotics, tranquilizers, medications for ulcers, heart disease and high blood pressure and anabolic steroids have all been shown to interfere with the libido and virility. So do alcohol and tobacco. Reducing or eliminating the use of these substances often repairs the problem. When discontinuing prescription drugs, be sure to work with an experienced healthcare professional to avoid complications.

In many cases, temporary impotence is caused by stress. A less hectic schedule and the use of relaxing herbs such as those listed for stress (see page 56) address this problem.

The herb ginseng is often called an aphrodisiac because its tonic properties help restore healthy function to all of the body's organs and systems (see page 64), aloe vera juice is a tonic beverage for which similar claims are made (see page 28) and ginkgo, which improves blood circulation, has been shown to help men whose impotence is caused by blocked arteries (see page 37). The following herbs are often used in herbal blends for the prostate and urinary tract, and some have important uses elsewhere, but they are among the most widely promoted and/or effective herbs for enhancing male sexuality.

Damiana (*Turnera diffusa—aphrodisiaca*)

As its Latin name suggests, damiana has a long-standing reputation as an aphrodisiac. In addition, the leaves of this fragrant plant are considered an effective antidepressant, urinary antiseptic, mild laxative and tonic for the central nervous system, prostate gland and hormones. As a nerve tonic, it is often combined with oats or skullcap; for improved prostate function, it is blended with saw palmetto berry; and for urinary tract infections, it can be mixed with echinacea, cranberry juice, uva ursi and other astringent, cleansing herbs.

Is it really an aphrodisiac? Pharmacognosy professor Varro E. Tyler says no. In his *Honest Herbal,* he attributed damiana's modern reputation to the efforts of 19th century druggists who sold the extract "to improve the sexual ability of the enfeebled and aged." Damiana tinctures became wildly popular, but skeptics attributed their commercial success to their high alcohol content and the addition of other herbs, such as coca, the source of cocaine. After reviewing damiana's chemical constituents, Tyler dismissed the plant's reputation as an herbal hoax.

But according to James Green in *The Male Herbal,* damiana deserves its reputation. "Used to treat impotence, it possibly has a testosterone-like action," he wrote, "and it may work by strengthening the male system." Green mentions a damiana liqueur sold in Mexico which is reputed to be an aphrodisiac and adds, "I have a number of acquaintances who attest to this as fact." Whether it's damiana or the placebo effect at work, this herb's reputation as an aphrodisiac is taken seriously by many herbalists.

Nettle or **Stinging Nettle** (*Urticia dioica*)

As annoying as nettle can be in the garden, its benefits include essential minerals, antispasmodic action and blood cleansing properties. Nettle offers safe relief from asthma and hay fever allergies, eczema and other skin conditions, gout and other forms of arthritis. In addition, nettle is a specific for the kidneys, urinary tract and prostate gland. According to Pacific Northwest herbalist Ryan Drum, nettle is most effective when freshly harvested (use protective gloves) and puréed in a blender or food processor with a small amount of water, a procedure that destroys its sting while enhancing its assimilation.

Stinging nettle tea is traditionally massaged into the scalp to prevent hair loss and used as a final rinse after shampooing to improve the condition of dark hair.

When combined with green oats, stinging nettle is said to be an aphrodisiac and virility drug.

Oats and **Oatstraw** (*Avena sativa*)

"Feeling your oats" and "sowing your wild oats" may be quaint old phrases. . . . or they may be accurate reflections of this grain's dynamic effects. When Chinese carp were accidentally fed a blend of green oats and stinging nettle, their reproductive rate increased dramatically. Chinese researchers measured elevated hormone levels and verified that the fish were mating more aggressively and more often than previously.

Testing a blend of green oats and stinging nettle on themselves, the researchers reported more energy and potency. They next conducted a double-blind experiment in which nearly 200 men took the mixture for several weeks. Ninety percent of the subjects reported an increased libido and improved performance.

Subsequent research in Europe and the U.S. has shown that athletes taking green oats and stinging nettle increased their aerobic capacity, muscle strength and testosterone levels, horses increased their stamina and endurance, and sexually dysfunctional men improved their performance.

Both young (green) and mature (golden) oatgrass and seeds are a nutritive tonic for the nervous system, recommended for nervous exhaustion, irritability, stress and overwork. Often blended with chamomile, lemon balm and other relaxing herbs, oats and oatgrass are made into teas, tinctures and capsules for frazzled nerves and the treatment of insomnia. In addition, oat bran and oat cereals are significant sources of dietary fiber that help reduce cholesterol levels, and oat baths have long been prescribed for sunburned skin, psoriasis, eczema and related conditions.

Yohimbe Bark (*Pausinystalia yohimba*)

The most famous herbal aphrodisiac, yohimbe, long used by native Africans for that purpose, is also the most controversial. Its list of alleged side effects reads like the warning notice on a prescription drug label. According to Varro Tyler, yohimbe is a monoamine oxidase inhibitor, which means that users should avoid foods such as liver, cheese and red wine, which contain tyramine, and diet aids containing phenylpropanolamine while taking yohimbe products. The herb should not be taken by anyone suffering from low blood pressure, diabetes, heart disease, liver disease or kidney disease or by anyone taking tranquilizers, narcotics, antihistamines or large quantities of alcohol. Yohimbe has been shown to produce anxiety and similar psychological reactions; in cases of schizophrenia, it may actually activate psychoses. Some researchers claim the herb is harmful when used to treat impotence caused by prostate inflammation or chronic inflammatory disease affecting the organs of reproduction. "These unpleasant and potentially hazardous reactions make it impossible to recommend the use of yohimbe for self-treatment," Tyler concluded.

Health warnings notwithstanding, yohimbe and its active ingredient, yohimbine, enjoy an undying reputation as sexual stimulants, reputations that may be well-deserved. Yohimbe extracts dilate the skin's blood vessels, lower blood pressure and stimulate reflex excitability in the lower regions of the spinal cord. In 1984, an experiment involving male rats showed that small doses of the herb increased their sexual arousal. Previous experiments, which used larger doses, produced other behavioral changes in test animals, suggesting that small quantities of the herb may produce the most impressive results.

To prepare a decoction, simmer 2 Tbs. yohimbe bark in 2 cups water for 10 minutes. James Green suggests adding 1 gram (1000 mg) of ascorbic acid (vitamin C) to the decoction to help avoid nausea and improve the herb's assimilation. Drink 1 to 2 cups approximately one hour before needed, once daily for a maximum of two weeks. If using a tincture, place 1 to 3 tsp. in a cup and add boiling water to evaporate most of the alcohol before using. Follow the same schedule as for the decoction described above.

Several products for athletes contain yohimbe; see page 27.

Because so little is known about yohimbe's safety, long-term side effects and effectiveness in humans, please observe the precautions listed above and consider this an herb to experiment with in small doses for short periods—if at all.

HERBS FOR ARTHRITIS

While no herb can reverse or cure arthritis in someone who eats all the wrong foods and avoids all the right ones, certain herbs work well in combination with dietary changes and active exercise to relieve, stop the progress of and even reverse inflammatory illnesses including osteoarthritis, rheumatism, gout and ankylosing spondylitis. For more information, see my book *Herbs for Arthritis*. Meanwhile, consider trying any or all of the following herbs.

Alfalfa (*Medicago sativa*)

This familiar field crop is an unusually rich source of minerals, for its tap roots extend 20 feet or more, absorbing nutrients that other plants can't reach. Alfalfa helps lower cholesterol and improve the blood's clotting ability; it is also a mild diuretic. A traditional therapy for arthritis, gout, rheumatism, fluid retention, peptic ulcers and digestive problems, alfalfa has demonstrated antibacterial, antifungal and antitumor activity in laboratory tests.

Cherries and Berries

Cherries, hawthorn berries, blueberries, grapes and other dark red-blue berries are rich sources of compounds that improve collagen metabolism and reduce joint inflammation. The famous botanist Linnaeus reportedly cured his gout by eating large quantities of strawberries morning and night, which led him to call them a "blessing of the gods." More recently, a gout "strawberry cure" of eating nothing but strawberries for several days was made popular by a French herbalist. Cherries are another specific for gout. During summer months, when these fruits are abundant, try to eat at least 1/2 cup daily, preferably more. If you prepare fresh juices, add them to your juicer as often as possible. People have derived results from canned, frozen, bottled, dried and even candied cherries, but for best results, make fresh fruit your first choice.

Feverfew (*Tanacetum parthenium*)

Best known as a treatment for preventing migraine headaches, feverfew is also effective in treating arthritis and other inflammatory illnesses. Feverfew's extremely bitter taste has made capsules and tablets more popular than teas, tinctures or fresh leaves. Note that a small percentage of those who try feverfew experience throat and mouth irritation. If you have an allergic reaction, discontinue use. For a review of this plant's practical applications, see *Feverfew: Your Headache May Be Over* by Ken Hancock.

Sarsaparilla (*Smilax officinalis*)

An important blood cleanser, general tonic, mild stimulant, diuretic and carminative (gas-relieving) herb, sarsaparilla is used in formulas that treat arthritis, gout, fluid retention, urinary tract infections, prostate problems, indigestion and flatulence. Brew sarsaparilla tea as a decoction, simmering 1 Tbs. dried root in 2 cups water for 10 to 15 minutes; let stand a few minutes, then strain and serve. Hot sarsaparilla tea rapidly expels gas from the stomach and intestines. Drink 1 to 2 cups tea or take ½ to 1 tsp. tincture daily.

Yucca (*Yucca baccata* and other species)

Yucca's saponin content makes it a friend to arthritics, for it reduces stress and swelling in the joints. Over 60 percent of patients tested with yucca supplements experienced diminished pain, swelling and stiffness; in addition, their blood pressure and cholesterol levels dropped, and intestinal toxicity improved as well. Yucca has no known side effects.

The standard dosage for yucca supplements is 2 tablets or capsules taken 3 times per day with meals. Liquid yucca extracts usually have a bitter, acrid taste improved by diluting the drops in fruit juice. Results are usually apparent within three weeks, with maximum improvement after four months.

HERBS FOR ATHLETES

Every health food store in America devotes at least a few shelves to nutritional supplements that promise athletes increased stamina, endurance and muscle strength.

Some of these products imply that they are natural sources of anabolic steroids, drugs that dramatically build muscle and physical strength. Despite their illegal status and adverse side effects, which include physical deformation, liver damage, impotence, sterility and psychological dysfunction, anabolic steroids are widely used because they work. Any herb promoted as a safe, natural, legal substitute has a ready market.

No plant produces anabolic steroids, so no herb can duplicate the effects of these drugs. However, several herbs contain steroidal saponins which are called anabolic steroid precursors, building blocks the body uses to create its own steroids and growth hormones. The difference is that a body ingesting synthetic steroids expands beyond its normal limits, while a body ingesting steroidal saponins cannot. No athlete taking a product containing yohimbe, wild yam, sarsaparilla, licorice root, damiana, yucca root, saw palmetto berry, ginseng root or Siberian ginseng, all of which contain anabolic steroid precursors, will experience the effects—or the side effects—that he would from synthetic steroids. But these herbs provide important nutritional support to any athlete who wants to improve his aerobic capacity, muscle development, physical strength, endurance and stamina.

It is worth noting that some products are made with adulterated herbs—inexpensive substitutes for ingredients such as ginseng, Siberian ginseng or yohimbe, or inferior sources of the real thing. Anyone shopping for the right athletic supplements should read product labels with the proverbial grain of salt. To test herbs containing anabolic steroid precursors, consider blending your own supplement with the help of a knowledgeable herbalist, and buy your herbs from a reliable, reputable source.

Tea tree oil (see page 50) is important to athletes because it treats cuts, burns, scrapes and sprains as well as athlete's foot, jock itch and toenail fungus. In addition, the following herbs are of special interest to athletes.

Aloe Vera (*Aloe vera*)

Best known for its skin soothing properties, the healing gel of aloe vera is a specific for burns, scalds, sunburn, skin infections, insect bites, cuts, wounds and abrasions. Simply break open the leaf and apply the cool, transparent gel. Rich in allantoin, a cell growth stimulant, aloe speeds healing and forms a protective bandage as it dries.

The bitter yellow inner rind of aloe vera is a harsh laxative, but when that irritating ingredient is filtered out or diluted, aloe vera juice or gel can be taken internally to improve digestion, increase stamina, boost immunity, fight infection and reduce the inflammation of arthritis, rheumatism or gout. According to Dr. Morton Walker in his book *Sexual Nutrition,* ''In its pure form, aloe vera is an excellent aphrodisiacal drink.'' He attributes its effects on the libido to its abundant vitamins, minerals, amino acids, essential oils and other nutrients.

Aloe vera juices are sold in health food stores. Look for brands containing mucopolysaccharides and natural preservatives such as vitamin C (ascorbic acid).

Arnica (*Arnica montana*)

Whether you're a weekend athlete, serious jogger or couch potato, arnica belongs in your medicine cabinet. Even better, carry arnica tincture with you whenever you work out or play competitive sports. Once baseball's standard remedy for bruises and sprains, this perennial herb with yellow blossoms is enjoying a revival. Its flowers have been used for centuries to make healing poultices, liniments, salves and lotions. Arnica is known as a ''specific'' or primary treatment for bruises and sprains. It also relieves the inflammation of phlebitis, rheumatic pain and related conditions.

Note: Arnica should not be taken internally except as a

homeopathic remedy, as it contains ingredients that stress the heart.

In *Medicinal Plants of the Pacific West,* Michael Moore wrote,

> Arnica works by stimulating and dilating blood vessels, particularly the specialized capillaries that control whether blood is piped into the small peripheral capillary beds or is shunted over to small veins, bypassing more widespread blood dispersal. Good, diffused blood transport and circulation into injured, bruised, or inflamed tissues helps speed up resolution and removal of waste products. Arnica does not have the anesthesia of menthol or wintergreen or the counterirritation property of other aromatic balms and should not be expected to have their immediate effects. Instead, in a few hours or overnight, it aids in removing the congestion that results from a bruise, sprain or hyperextension.

I'm fond of arnica tincture because it stopped the sharp pain so dramatically after hitting my elbow really hard on the corner of a desk. I was able to splash on a generous amount of arnica tincture within one minute and the pain truly stopped immediately; so did the swelling and bruising. Timing is everything, for similar bruises treated hours after the injury have been slower to heal and stop hurting.

Like arnica tincture, arnica massage oil is effective in the treatment of wounds, sprains, bruises and joint inflammation.

In some cases, the frequent application of arnica results in skin irritation, in which case its use should be reduced.

Wild Yam (*Dioscorea villosa*)

Best known as the source of birth control pills, wild yam root contains hormone precursors with an action similar to that of cortisone. In recent years wild yam creams have become popular among women, whose menopausal or menstrual symptoms are relieved by the natural progesterone their skin absorbs.

But wild yam creams, as well as capsules, teas and tinctures, help treat glandular imbalances, arthritis, joint injuries, intestinal spasms and prostate problems in men. Among the benefits claimed by users of wild yam creams are hair growth reversing male pattern baldness, improved libido, weight loss, a more youthful appearance and increased endurance and stamina.

Although widely quoted by promoters and manufacturers, the claims made for wild yam creams are controversial, for none have been proved in clinical trials and neither has the product's safety. It is true that some physicians have prescribed wild yam creams for years without observing harmful side effects, but most of their patients are women; the use of the cream by men is not as well-documented.

To use wild yam as a tea, brew a decoction by simmering 1 tsp. dried root in 2 cups water for 10 to 15 minutes. Wild yam combines well with marshmallow root, ginger and chamomile for relief from indigestion and intestinal cramping. It can be blended with black cohosh and other antispasmodic herbs for rheumatism, arthritis and to speed the healing of sprains and other injuries.

HERBS FOR CIRCULATION AND THE HEART

Blood pressure, cholesterol, heart disease and circulatory problems affect most American men. The following herbs help improve circulation, lower blood pressure and lower cholesterol levels, but they can't repair the damage created by an unhealthy diet or sedentary lifestyle. A low-fat diet based on fresh fruits and vegetables; vitamin, mineral and trace mineral supplements; large quantities of drinking water; the use of unrefined sea salt rather than refined table salt and regular active exercise all improve the heart and circulatory system. For a more comprehensive review of plant-based therapies, see my book *Herbs for the Heart*.

Because stress management is so important to heart health, see also the section describing herbs for stress (page 56).

One of the most versatile medicinal herbs is garlic, described on page 62 as a tonic for all of the body's systems. Research has repeatedly shown that garlic has a healing effect on the heart and circulation. In addition to the following herbs, consider adding garlic to your daily diet, either as the pungent cooking herb or in capsules. Both raw and cooked garlic have been shown to reduce harmful cholesterol levels, reduce high blood pressure and improve blood flow.

Bilberry (*Vaccinum myrtillus*)

The bilberry, a shrubby perennial plant that grows in the northeast United States and Europe, is commonly known as the wild blueberry, dyeberry, huckleberry, hurtleberry, whinberry, whortleberry or wineberry. Bilberry has become popular in recent years because of its ability to repair and improve the capillaries. When impaired, these fragile blood vessels can be linked to high blood pressure, atherosclerosis, diabetes, stroke, heart attack or blindness caused by damage to the retina. Less dramatic but still serious are the links between weak capillaries and bruising, varicose veins, "spider" veins, susceptibility to cold temperatures, poor night vision and numbness in the legs and feet.

Bilberries contain anthocyanins, flavonoid compounds that color the berries' juice and skin. These compounds are antioxidants, which protect cells from the damage caused by free radicals. Free radicals are fragments of chemicals that can damage membranes and destroy cells, but capillaries protected by bilberry's flavonoids are able to stretch, increasing blood flow and oxygenation.

Research has shown that bilberry extracts not only strengthen capillaries and prevent bruising and hemorrhage, they reduce calcium plaque deposits in blood vessels, commonly called hardening of the arteries or atherosclerosis. Because bilberry thins the blood, it protects the circulatory system against clotting. In fact, bilberry strengthens the capillaries so effectively that in Europe it is used to prevent bleeding during and after surgery. Patients are treated for 10 days prior to surgery as a preventive measure.

In America, bilberry is best known for its ability to protect the eyes. During World War II, British pilots ate bilberry preserves to improve their eyesight, especially their night vision. Research has confirmed bilberry's effectiveness in this regard; not only does it reduce the amount of time the eye needs to adapt to darkness after exposure to bright light, it can significantly improve vision, probably because it improves blood circulation within the eye.

Less familiar to Americans are bilberry's anticancer properties and its ability to prevent ulcers. The herb's flavonoids apparently increase mucus secretion in the stomach, which protects its lining from hyperacidity and from the adverse side effects of aspirin, other drugs and alcohol.

Cayenne or **Chile Peppers** (*Capsicum annuum*)

Hot peppers bring the dullest dish to life, warm the mind and body—and when you swallow an unusually hot specimen, choke on the fumes of a freshly cut jalapeno or, even worse, touch your eye after chopping one, they can be the most irritating vegetables on the planet. No wonder their name derives from the Greek word meaning "to bite."

How hot is hot? For many years the capsaicin content of peppers has been measured on a scale of 0 for sweet bell peppers to 350,000 for habañero or Scotch bonnet peppers. Ten thousand heat units is mildly spicy and 50,000 units tastes hot to most American palates. Anything over 100,000 is seriously hot.

Only recently have scientists discovered how healing peppers are. Taken internally, they improve digestion, increase circulation and enhance memory. Applied externally, they speed healing, though the initial application may sting. Cayenne peppers contain more vitamin C than any fruit, and they practically define Mexican cooking.

Cayenne has received much publicity in recent years through the efforts of Dick Quinn, author of the book *Left for Dead*. After experiencing a heart attack, unsuccessful bypass surgery, debilitating side effects, fatigue and depression, Quinn was walking by a lake when he met the mother of a friend. She noticed he was exhausted after his short trip from the car and told him to begin taking cayenne red pepper right away.

"It seemed preposterous to recommend red pepper after what I'd been through," he wrote. "This was too serious for such nonsense." The woman had seen Dr. John Christopher, whose *School of Natural Healing* is a classic American herbal, at a seminar during which a man had a heart attack in the hotel lobby. In one of the most widely reported and dramatic demonstrations of herbal healing, Christopher sent a hotel employee to the kitchen for cayenne pepper and a glass of water, which he mixed and gave to the man. Within minutes, the heart attack victim was up and walking.

Dick Quinn didn't believe her. He knew that the man had something else wrong with him. Heart attacks don't disappear just because someone swallows hot peppers. He was lying on the sand trying to make sense of her ridiculous story when she said again, "You look terrible. You need capsicum—red cayenne pepper.'' To prove her wrong, he went home and followed his doctor's instructions to the letter. But instead of recovering, his arteries collapsed and he began moving in slow motion, fainting in inconvenient places and suffering terrible bouts of weakness. Then a blind spell occurred; his vision gradually disappeared until he could see nothing.

A few days after that episode, which slowly reversed itself, Quinn saw his cardiologist for a six-month checkup. The more he demanded answers, the more distant and defensive the doctor became. All he could recommend was another surgery. ''At that moment,'' Quinn wrote, ''I realized it was entirely up to me to heal myself. I knew nothing at all about treating heart disease, but I had to take charge. He was dropping me. He had done what he knew how to do and now he didn't have to care any more.'' His doctor had followed the accepted procedures. They didn't work, but that was okay. The patient should now die quietly, without making a fuss.

The only alternative treatment Quinn had ever heard of was his friend's mother's recommendation, so in desperation he drove to a store and bought a can of powdered cayenne pepper for 69 cents. He went home, emptied some capsules from an old prescription, filled them with cayenne and swallowed three. Nothing happened and he went to bed.

When he awoke an hour earlier than usual, instead of being exhausted, he felt energetic. With mixed emotions, he walked outside. It was only after he had moved a ladder, carried a shovel and cleared the entire porch roof of snow that he realized something dramatic had happened and that it was linked to the cayenne pepper. After that, Quinn discontinued all prescription drugs, including blood thinners and high blood pressure medication. Instead, he took three cayenne capsules a day and lived another lively, energetic 18 years.

If you decide to try cayenne capsules, be sure to take them with food and plenty of water, tea or juice; cayenne taken on an empty stomach with small amounts of liquid can burn for hours. However, even this side effect disappears with regular use. If you'd like to reduce or eliminate your use of prescription drugs, work with a health care professional.

Cayenne heals ulcers (bland rather than spicy foods used to be recommended for ulcer patients, but cayenne works better), stops hemorrhaging, speeds the healing of wounds, eases congestion, improves digestion and elimination, reduces pain, warms cold hands and feet, relieves swelling in varicose veins and hemorrhoids, helps prevent colds and flu and prevents the spread of infection. Although some who suffer from rheumatism and arthritis are sensitive to members of the nightshade family (tomatoes, potatoes, eggplant, tobacco and peppers), those who are not derive significant pain relief from cayenne pepper and from massage oils containing cayenne. It relieves pain so effectively that researchers at Yale University developed a chile pepper taffy for patients with painful mouth lesions resulting from cancer therapy.

Ginkgo (*Ginkgo biloba*)

Botanists tell us that the ginkgo, also known as the maidenhair tree, is the oldest tree species on earth, having survived an estimated 200 million years. Common in Europe and North America during the Age of Dinosaurs, the ginkgo disappeared during the last Ice Age from all of its native habitats except China, where it continued to thrive and where its healing properties were recognized long ago.

Male ginkgo trees are ornamental, while female trees produce a foul-smelling fruit at maturity. The fruit contains a nut which is a delicacy in Chinese cooking. Both male and female trees produce leaves whose medicinal properties have generated a flurry of scientific research.

In China, ginkgo leaves were traditionally used as a brain tonic, to relieve asthma symptoms and to treat coughs, filariasis (a chronic disease caused by parasitic nematodes) and diarrhea. Externally, ginkgo was used to treat skin sores and freckles and a decoction of boiled leaves is still used for frostbite.

Today's ginkgo research focuses on the plant's ability to treat asthma, toxic shock, Alzheimer's disease and various circulatory disorders. It has repeatedly been shown to increase the flow of blood through aging vessels, especially in the brain. This explains its effectiveness in the treatment and prevention of problems as varied as asthma, hearing loss (cochlear deafness), stroke, heart attack, dementia, depression, tinnitus (ringing in the ears), fatigue, vision problems such as macular degeneration, high blood pressure, kidney problems, allergies, brain function impairment, memory loss, dizziness, impotence and poor circulation. Many hundreds of papers have been published in scientific and medical journals around the world reporting on laboratory tests and clinical trials examining ginkgo preparations.

Gingko's active constituents are present in the leaves just as they change from green to yellow in the fall. They consist of flavonoid glycosides and ginkgolides, both of which prevent inflammation and blood clotting. In most extraction processes, dried ginkgo leaves are ground and mixed with organic solvents that release their chemical compounds. The blend is heated and the process repeated several times before further refining, which results in an extract with a 24 percent concentration of flavonoids believed by European pharmaceutical researchers to be the optimum therapeutic concentration. However, whole ginkgo leaves remain a popular ingredient in medicinal tea and tincture blends for which many herbalists report good results and few side effects.

Because it interferes with blood clotting, ginkgo should not be taken by those with clotting disorders. Some users, after taking extremely large amounts, have reported restlessness, irritability, diarrhea, vomiting and nausea. The recommended dosages are considered nontoxic.

Most experts agree that ginkgo preparations have to be taken consistently for two to four months before significant results are noticed. Gingko leaves are often mixed with gotu kola (another memory-enhancing herb) in tea blends, tinctures and memory tonics. The medicinal constituents of ginkgo do not dissolve readily in water, which is why, unlike most leaves, they should be boiled as a decoction. To brew a memory tonic tea containing equal parts of ginkgo, gotu kola and the culinary herb rosemary, first simmer 1 Tbsp. ginko in 2 cups water for 10 to 15 minutes. Remove from heat, add 1 Tbsp. each of gotu kola and rosemary, cover and let stand an additional 10 minutes.

For men, ginkgo is of special interest because it has been shown to cure impotence caused by blocked arteries. In one study, 50 patients with arterial erectile impotence were treated with 240 mg of ginkgo extract daily and all reported significantly improved erections; in another, 60 men who did not respond to injections of the erection-boosting drug papaverine took 60 mg of ginkgo extract daily and half regained potency within six months.

Gotu Kola (*Centella asiatica*)

The round, fan-shaped leaves of gotu kola grow close to the ground in a thick green carpet. In tropical climates, it is a familiar lawn and roadside weed. Known to Indian writers centuries ago as an herb that increases longevity, gotu kola traveled with people from that country as they settled in the Caribbean, Hawaii and other warm climates. Now recognized as an important herb for the circulatory system, gotu kola is cultivated around the world for its medicinal benefits.

If you do not already grow gotu kola as a garden or house plant, consider doing so. Much of the gotu kola sold commercially is of poor quality, so your own plant is insurance of excellence. Fresh gotu kola has a pleasant, spicy or tangy taste in teas and salads. Gotu kola is easy to grow indoors in winter, outdoors in summer and outdoors all year in warm climates.

The name gotu kola may derive from the plant's Sinhalese name, *hingotu kola,* but this is uncertain. Its common names include centella and Indian pennywort; its Sanskrit name is *brahmi*. It is not related to the kola nut, which contains caffeine; gotu kola does not.

Research has shown that a water extract of fresh gotu kola leaves increased the learning response of laboratory rats, and two studies of developmentally disabled children showed a significant increase in mental abilities. Gotu kola is used in memory tonics designed for students of all ages, for the elderly and for people in high stress jobs who have to think and respond quickly.

In addition to its uses as a mental stimulator, gotu kola has important benefits in skin healing. Modern research on the plant began in 1949 when scientists in Madagascar injected an extract of gotu kola directly into leprosy nodules, perforated ulcers and lesions on the eyes and fingers of leprosy patients and observed rapid healing. This led to additional studies using gotu kola extracts, teas, poultices and injections to heal skin lesions, burns and different types of wounds, all with significant results.

During the last 20 years, scientists have studied the effects of gotu kola on not only mental function and skin disorders but heart disease, inflammatory illnesses, circulatory problems such as phlebitis, fluid retention and surgical wounds. It is said to improve sports performance and has a following among athletes.

Gotu kola's only known side effect is a skin rash in sensitive individuals. The recommended dose for tea (1 tsp. dried herb infused in 1 cup boiling water) is up to 2 cups per day. Gotu kola is often combined with other herbs.

Guggulow or **Gum Guggul** (*Commiphor mukul*)

A tree resin widely used in Europe and its native India, guggulow helps normalize body weight and blood cholesterol levels. Research shows it to have few side effects; an estimated one percent of capsule users have an allergic reaction and should discontinue use. A mild thyroid tonic, guggulow helps balance the metabolism, reduce obesity and prevent heart attacks.

Hawthorn Berries (*Crataegus oxyacantha*)

Also called the hawmay, mayblossom, mayflower, maythorn or whitethorn, the hawthorn has nearly 1,000 species in North America. Hawthorn belongs to the family *rosaceae,* whose members include the rose, peach, almond, apple and strawberry. Its name comes from the sharp thorns on its twiggy branches.

The fruit, flowers and leaves of the hawthorn have been used to treat heart diseases for hundreds of years. Modern science has confirmed such use by demonstrating that hawthorn berries dilate blood vessels, allowing blood to circulate more efficiently and lowering blood pressure. Hawthorn also improves the heart itself, acting directly on the heart muscle to help heal damage and improve the organ's operation.

Unlike prescription drugs prescribed for heart ailments,

hawthorn berries appear to be safe and free from adverse side effects.

Botanical drugs are widely used in Europe, where the clinical testing of plant-based medicines is common. In 1953, scientists in Germany measured an 83 percent increase in coronary blood flow following the intravenous administration of hawthorn extract. Later research has shown that hawthorn preparations taken orally increase blood flow to the brain. A study conducted in 1984 demonstrated that hawthorn tablets reduced the pain of angina by 84 percent, compared to a placebo's 37 percent reduction. Of the 29 patients involved in this study, 13 stopped taking nitroglycerine tablets altogether, while another 10 were able to reduce their intake of nitroglycerine. In 1987 another study showed hawthorn extract to be an effective peripheral vasodilator in a placebo-controlled double-blind study on older patients suffering from angina pectoris.

Despite its effectiveness, hawthorn is not well-known in the United States. Some speculate that the reason is hawthorn's lack of exotic drama: it isn't rare and its effects are not so dramatic as other botanical drugs, such as the digitalis preparations made from foxglove. Hawthorn works slowly and subtly to improve circulation and heart function.

Among the conditions for which hawthorn preparations are recommended are irregular heartbeat, geriatric or stressed heart, hypertension, coronary insufficiency, myocardism following contagious disease, sensitivity to cardiac glycosides, cerebral circulatory disturbances, heart attack, heart failure, damage to the coronary arteries and angina pectoris. Hawthorn is a mild sedative, making it useful in cases of heart disease linked to nervousness and stress. It does not lead to dependence and can be taken in large doses without harm. In fact, it is important to give a sufficiently large dose daily for at least three months and up to several years, as needed, because hawthorn's effect is not cumulative.

Hawthorn berry preparations are considered safe to use in combination with pharmaceutical drugs such as digitoxin, and in many cases its use allows the patient to reduce or eliminate the use of such drugs. Of course, such substitutions should be made under a physician's supervision.

In Germany, where over three dozen hawthorn-based heart medications are available, one teaspoon of hawthorn tincture on arising and another before bed is the standard recommendation. Because the taste is bitter, hawthorn can be mixed with honey, lemon, stevia or other herbs to improve its taste. In addition to its cardiovascular benefits, hawthorn berry is an excellent source of vitamin C. Hawthorn berry jams and jellies are popular wherever the plant grows wild, and the berries can be made into a fresh tincture or dried and made into a tea or tincture, as can the flowers and leaves. To make your own effective hawthorn berry tincture, follow the procedure described on page 55.

Herbs for Colds, Flu and Chronic Coughs

If you feel the symptoms of an oncoming cold, or if the flu is going around and you want to boost your immunity, review the infection-fighting herbs on pages 48 to 51. Astragalus, echinacea and grapefruit seed extract are all effective if taken at the beginning of an infectious disease, and when everyone around you is sick, taking these herbs will help keep you well.

For sore throats and coughs, licorice root (page 44), ginger root (page 43), ginkgo (page 35) and garlic (page

62) are traditional therapies. So are gargles made of salt water or salted teas made of the culinary herbs sage, thyme and rosemary. Hot lemonade, hot baths, facial steam treatments (see page 74), freshly made fruit and vegetable juices and hot soups containing garlic, chile peppers and other warming spices are all beneficial.

Grindelia or **Gumweed** (*Grindelia spp.*)

An antispasmodic and expectorant, grindelia is most useful in treating chronic bronchial coughs and infections as well as allergies such as hay fever. Externally, the plant or its tea can be applied to poison ivy or poison oak rashes and insect bites. A mild sedative, grindelia helps lower blood pressure and reduce a fast pulse. It is sometimes combined with licorice root. Because grindelia can irritate the kidneys, it should be taken in small doses and for short periods of time, not every day for months.

Horehound (*Marribium vulgare*)

Once a popular candy ingredient, horehound's bitter leaves are an effective expectorant, helping clear the lungs of fluid and mucus. If you can find them, keep old fashioned horehound drops on hand for acute and chronic coughs, or brew an infusion of equal parts horehound, peppermint and fresh grated ginger. Drink up to 3 cups daily. In large quantities, horehound has a laxative effect.

HERBS FOR DIGESTION, HEARTBURN, ULCERS

If the billions of dollars Americans spend on ulcer medications, antacids, heartburn preparations, gas relievers and prescription drugs for irritable bowel syndrome, diverticulitis and other symptoms of indigestion are an accurate indication, most of us suffer after every meal.

Much of our discomfort stems directly from the foods we eat, which are usually overprocessed, stripped of nutrients, low in fiber, high in fats that are difficult to digest and otherwise deficient. For a review of appropriate dietary changes and herbs that support them, see my book *Herbs for Improved Digestion.*

All of the tonic herbs (page 61) and herbs that improve circulation (page 30) are helpful because they increase the flow of digestive fluids, improve the flow of blood and support all of the body's organs. In addition, the following are considered specifics for digestion.

Ginger (*Zingiber officinale*)

The familiar culinary spice can be used fresh or dried, in teas, capsules, tablets, tinctures or in foods, alone or in combination with other herbs, to treat digestive disorders, improve circulation and prevent nausea. To prevent motion sickness, take enough powdered ginger in capsules (as many as 6 or 8) to cause a mild heartburn sensation, half an hour to an hour before setting sail or taking off. In tests, ginger outperformed Dramamine, a motion sickness drug that, unlike ginger, causes drowsiness. On long flights or ocean cruises, repeat as needed every 4 to 6 hours.

Like other aromatic herbs and spices, ginger helps prevent and relieve flatulence and other symptoms of digestive distress. A catalyst or stimulant herb, ginger is often added to tea blends to improve the performance of other ingredients.

Lemon Balm or **Balm** (*Melissa officinalis*)

This cheerful mint with a pronounced lemon fragrance is one of the world's favorite herbs. Revered throughout Europe for its antispasmodic and carminative (gas-relieving) properties, lemon balm is a common ingredient in after-dinner digestive aids such as melissa water or melissa tincture. It is often combined with chamomile and peppermint, which have similar properties.

Lemon balm is used in Europe as a topical remedy for both cold sores and genital herpes. In a 1994 study of 115 patients suffering from cold sores, 60 percent had complete healing after four days of applying a melissa cream five times daily. After six days, 87 percent were healed and after eight days, 96 percent were healed. Cold sores usually last 10 to 14 days without treatment. A strong (medicinal strength) infusion of lemon balm can be applied as a wash several times daily to speed the healing of genital herpes.

Licorice Root (*Glycyrrhiza glabra*)

Most familiar as an ingredient in black candy ropes and other confections, licorice root is so sweet and aromatic that it's often used to flavor herbal teas. Because of its relaxing effect on the digestive tract, especially the stomach, it is an effective treatment for ulcers. It is also recommended for adrenal exhaustion, stress, hypoglycemia, chronic fatigue, sore throats and chronic coughs.

Unfortunately, untreated licorice has side effects. Glycyrrhizin, its most active principle, can cause edema (fluid retention), heartburn, and, in some people, headaches. It should not be taken by those with high blood pressure. These side effects are well-documented in German medical texts, for licorice has long been prescribed by that country's physicians for ulcers and stomach pain. One common result of daily licorice overconsumption is a round moon face caused by fluid retention.

In Europe, licorice roots are now treated to remove their glycyrrhizin content, but in the U.S. and Canada, the roots are sold untreated. You can, however, purchase deglycyrrhizinated licorice capsules, tinctures and other preparations in health food stores. Because of its effectiveness, deglycyrrhizinated licorice is beginning to appear in over-the-counter products for the treatment of heartburn and acid indigestion.

To use licorice for therapeutic purposes, such as the treatment of ulcers or to prevent anxiety and stress or repair the adrenal glands, it is better to take deglycyrrhizined licorice than to drink large quantities of strongly brewed licorice tea. A daily cup of beverage-strength licorice root tea isn't likely to cause problems, but several cups per day could do so in sensitive people. In small doses and for occasional use, or when used as a gargle for sore throats or tired vocal cords, adverse side effects are unlikely.

Marshmallow Root (*Althaea officinalis*)

A soothing, demulcent plant with diuretic properties, marshmallow is an important nutritive tonic and digestive aid. Rich in vegetable mucilage and easily assimilated calcium, marshmallow root is a common ingredient in herbal blends designed to treat digestive, urinary, prostate, respiratory and inflammatory conditions. Because its essential oils are fragile and volatile, many herbalists recommend that marshmallow root tea be made as a cold infusion. Pour 2 cups cold water over 1 Tbsp. finely chopped dried root and let stand overnight without heating.

Peppermint (*Mentha piperita*) and Spearmint (*Mentha aquatica*)

These versatile culinary mints have important digestive applications. They are among the most effective carminative agents, relieving flatulence and indigestion. Peppermint helps prevent nausea, promotes liver and gallbladder function, alleviates spasms and gently disinfects the digestive tract. The German authority Rudolf Fritz Weiss notes that peppermint is not recommended for ulcers because it is not an anti-inflammatory agent and, because frequent use lessens its effectiveness, peppermint is not recommended for extended use on a daily basis.

Because hydrochloric acid and other digestive secretions prevent peppermint oil from reaching the intestines, it has no value in the treatment of diverticulitis or irritable bowel syndrome unless the essential oil is protected by capsules designed to break down in the intestines rather than in the stomach. Enteric-coated peppermint capsules are widely used in Europe with much success for these conditions. Similar products are beginning to be sold in the U.S.; check with your health food store or pharmacy.

If you are taking homeopathic preparations, bear in mind that mint is said to interfere with the effectiveness of homeopathy. Most practitioners advise their patients to avoid mint tea and mint flavored products, such as chewing gum, toothpaste and mouthwash, while taking homeopathic drugs.

Swedish Bitters

The late Austrian herbalist Maria Treben made Swedish bitters a household name in Europe after she discovered its recipe in an old manuscript. The recipe appears in her book *Health Through God's Pharmacy*. The tincture has far too many uses to list here, ranging from the treatment of stomach cramps, ulcers and indigestion to external application for wounds and insect bites. It's no exaggeration to say that Treben found 100 effective uses for this tincture, which she credited with saving her life. Though not the worst-tasting liquid you'll ever encounter, Swedish bitters lives up to its name and it's an acquired taste: strong, pungent, and yes, very bitter.

Containing myrrh, saffron, rhubarb root, carline thistle root, angelica root and other aromatic, bitter constituents, Swedish bitters is the most effective digestive tonic I have found—especially when made at home and allowed to age longer than the commercial product sold in health food stores. Men who can't get through the day without antacids or prescription ulcer drugs find that a teaspoon of Swedish bitters before meals leaves them free of heartburn, gastric upset and even the worst symptoms of indigestion. Many are able to reduce or eliminate medication altogether.

The Austrian distributor of Maria Treben Swedish Bitters ships the dry Swedish bitters blend to U.S. customers at a reasonable price; each box makes over a quart of Swedish bitters tincture. To order, see the Appendix. As this product is not distributed in the U.S. or England, there is no English language labeling, so save these instructions:

> Add 5 cups of 80-proof vodka to the contents of one box in a large glass jar. Any distilled liquor of at least 80-proof will work well; substitute rum or brandy as desired. Seal the jar tightly and leave it in a warm place, shaking it every few days. Treben recommended letting the jar stand for 14 days, but the blend's flavor and intensity increase substantially if you leave it for four weeks or longer. Do so for best results. To use, strain the tincture through cheesecloth and store it in tightly closed amber glass bottles away from heat and light. Properly stored, the tincture will keep indefinitely.

To use Swedish bitters for improved digestion, take 1 teaspoon diluted with water or straight from the spoon a few minutes before each meal. For best results, hold the bitters on your tongue for 20 seconds or more before swallowing. It takes getting used to, but the benefits are often dramatic. For indigestion after eating, repeat as needed.

HERBS THAT FIGHT INFECTION

Whether it's a cold, the flu or a sore that won't heal, infection-fighting herbs boost the immune system and help control opportunistic pathogens. Sometimes called herbal antibiotics, these plants are often more effective than their pharmaceutical counterparts, for antibiotics have no effect on viruses, and many bacteria are now drug-resistant.

One of the best infection-fighting herbs is garlic, described in detail on page 62. Garlic's antimicrobial action is strongest in raw garlic and aged garlic extracts, but even cooked garlic contains some infection-fighting ingredients.

Astragalus (*Astragalus membranaceous*)

One of the most popular Chinese herbs, astragalus root is revered as a powerful immune system strengthener. Traditionally used to treat anxiety and fatigue, astragalus has general tonic properties; that is, it heals, repairs and supports the entire body, increasing stamina and building resistance to disease and infection. Its diuretic properties make it a specific for the kidneys and urinary tract; it is also recommended for conditions relating to the spleen, lungs and blood. In lab tests, astragalus has been shown to kill viruses, destroy cancer cells and induce interferon production.

Astragalus root can be brewed as a decoction (simmer 1 Tbs. dried root in 2 cups water for 10 to 15 minutes, let stand 5 minutes, strain and serve; drink 1 or 2 cups daily), added to rice, soups or stews during cooking, or sautéed in honey to create a medicinal syrup. Astragalus is an excellent herb to take during outbreaks of colds and flu, while training for athletic events and in times of stress or overwork. It is available in tinctures and capsules and is also a popular ingredient in blends, especially those designed for the immune system. For everyday use as an immune-stimulating tonic, take 1 capsule 2 or 3 times daily or up to 1 teaspoon of tincture daily. To treat a cold, the flu or any acute infection, take up to 3 capsules 3 times daily or up to 1 teaspoon of tincture 3 times daily.

No dangerous side effects have been reported, but some astragalus users have experienced mild diarrhea or abdominal bloating. Reducing the dosage eliminates these symptoms.

Echinacea (*E. purpurea, E. angustifolia*)

One of America's best-selling herbs, the purple coneflower (*E. purpurea*) and its close cousin, the narrow-leaved coneflower (*E. angustifolia*), are often recommended for the treatment of colds and flu. Echinacea is most effective in combatting infections when taken in large doses in capsules or tincture for short periods, such as 1 cup of tea or 1 teaspoon tincture every hour for one or two days. For best results, use a tincture made from the fresh rather than dried plant; look for a dark color, sharp fragrance and pungent taste. The entire echinacea plant is medicinal, from dramatic blossom to leaf, stem, seed and roots.

Grapefruit Seed Extract or **Citrus Seed Extract**

Originally developed as a natural fungicide to preserve fresh fruits during shipping, grapefruit seed extract has become a popular alternative to antibiotic drugs and a widely tested disinfectant. Laboratory tests show that dilute solutions of the extract, which is extremely bitter tasting, kill infectious bacteria, viruses, molds, yeasts, parasites, fungi and other pathogens on contact.

The liquid extract added to lake or stream water in sufficient quantity to taste protects campers and hikers against *Giardia lamblia* and other waterborne contaminants. Travelers to foreign countries can take the debittered, powdered extract in capsules to prevent diarrhea and worm infestations. Dilute solutions of the liquid extract treat athlete's foot, jock itch, yeast infections, burns, rashes, ear infections and a variety of external conditions.

Tea Tree Oil (*Melaleuca alternifolia*)

An essential oil, tea tree oil is distilled from the tea tree, which grows in the swampy lowlands of New South Wales on Australia's northeast coast. Its distilled oil has a pleasant, distinctive, rather medicinal fragrance, and though it is gentle enough to use undiluted on adult skin, it is an antiseptic bactericide 12 times stronger than carbolic acid. A penetrating germicide and fungicide, it dissolves pus and debris without harming the skin.

Most people tolerate undiluted tea tree oil very well, but if your skin is very sensitive, try a "patch test" by placing a drop on the inside of your elbow and leaving it overnight. If undiluted tea tree oil irritates your skin, dilute it in an equal quantity of olive oil, or follow the instructions on page 74 to prepare a 15 percent tea tree oil solution in water.

Even in dilute solutions, tea tree oil kills on contact nearly all harmful bacteria, viruses, molds, yeast, fungi, parasites and other pathogens. Best known for its effective treatment of athlete's foot, jock itch and dandruff, tea tree oil has become a popular ingredient in toothpaste and mouthwash, for it helps prevent gum disease. In addition, tea tree oil is often added to herbal insect repellents, massage oils and sports rubs. Full strength or dilute solutions disinfect and heal infected wounds, boils, ingrown hairs, blisters, abrasions and burns. No wonder its Australian manufacturers call it a "medicine kit in a bottle."

See the uses of tea tree oil described in the aromatherapy section, pages 73–78. For more detailed information, see my booklet *Nature's Antiseptics: Tea Tree Oil and Grapefruit Seed Extract.*

Herbs for the Prostate

Many herbs help the prostate, including several described as aphrodisiacs (page 19) and those that repair the urinary tract (page 20). The following, which are considered specifics for the prostate, are the most widely recommended.

Self-treatment of prostate disorders should be approached with the understanding that the herbs described here do not cure prostate cancer. Work with a holistic physician or healthcare professional to be sure your condition can be treated by saw palmetto and other herbs. If you are taking a prescription drug such as Proscar, seek professional advice before discontinuing its use.

Cat's Claw or **Uña de Gato** (*Uncaria tomentosa*)

Cat's claw, known in Spanish as *uña de gato,* is a South American rain forest vine that grows over 100 feet in length with sharp, curving thorns that look like a cat's claws. For centuries, native Indians have used the vine's root to prepare a medicinal decoction to treat tumors and other serious diseases.

Thanks to the promotional efforts of its supporters, cat's claw has become a best-seller, a "cure-all" herb recommended for the treatment of illnesses as varied as cancer, prostatitis, digestive disorders, HIV/AIDS, bursitis, systemic candidiasis, diabetes, lupus, chronic fatigue syndrome, premenstrual syndrome, environmental toxin poisoning, chronic depression, immune system impairment, allergies and genital herpes. Does it work? There is at least one well-documented Peruvian case of cancer apparently cured by cat's claw, and its most enthusiastic advocate, Philip Steinberg, credits cat's claw tea with curing his long-term prostate inflammation. German research supports at least some of the claims made on its behalf, but cat's claw is among the least tested and least understood of the popular medicinal herbs. No clinical trials of cat's claw teas, extracts or capsules have been conducted to test its effectiveness, and critics charge that promoters misinterpreting laboratory test results have misrepresented the herb.

Product quality is a serious consideration, for another South American plant with the same common name has been sold as *Uncaria tomentosa,* and although only the root's bark was used in traditional medicine and tested in Europe, most of the cat's claw imported to the U.S. is the bark of the above-ground vine, not its root. As the rate of harvesting increases, the world's supply of cat's claw, especially its medicinal root, is in serious danger of extinction.

Cat's claw was unknown in North America until the early 1990s, so it has a short history of popular use here. The herb is said to be safe, and lab tests on rats have shown no toxicity. However, little is known about its long-term effects.

In addition to questioning the quality of cat's claw in capsules, the Austrian physician Klaus Keplinger, who has received patents for his cat's claw extracts, believes that the herb should never be taken raw, only cooked, which is its traditional method of preparation.

By the 21st century, when some predict that authentic cat's claw will be extinct or impossible to obtain, we may know the answers to the questions this exotic herb raises.

In the meantime, cat's claw might or might not be an effective therapy for the illness you hope to treat. According to Philip Steinberg, whose efforts have convinced thousands of American men to try the herb, his benign prostatic hypertrophy improved within a week of drinking 3 to 4 cups cat's claw decoction (simmered tea) daily. He now claims to be symptom-free.

Pumpkin Seeds, Pumpkin Seed Oil
(*Cucurbita pepo*)

The familiar Hallowe'en jack-o-lantern offers more than a goofy grin; its seeds are a traditional worming herb as well as an important food for the prostate. Pumpkin seeds are rich in zinc, linoleic acid (vitamin F) and vegetable mucilage. Both pumpkin seeds and pumpkin seed oil are used in prostate support formulas. Many holistic physicians recommend that their patients eat a handful of fresh pumpkin seeds daily.

Pygeum (*Pygeum africanum, Prunus africanum*)

The bark of this African shrub has been shown to be effective in the treatment of several prostate disorders, including benign prostatic hyperplasia, prostatitis and prostate-related sexual dysfunction. In an experimental double-blind study in Austria, patients receiving 50 mg twice daily for two months showed significant improvement in overall symptoms, and other studies have demonstrated improved urinary flow characteristics as well as improvement in sexual function. Pygeum's major side effects are unpleasant gastric symptoms such as nausea, vomiting, diarrhea and indigestion in up to 13 percent of those receiving it.

The standardized extract used in pygeum's double-blind, placebo-controlled studies is a commercially prepared solvent extract manufactured in Europe. Pygeum bark is not available as an herb in North America, but the extract is used in an increasing number of dietary supplements and herbal products sold here. It is often combined with saw palmetto berry and stinging nettle.

Pygeum has been shown in animal studies to have an anti-inflammatory and antiedema effect. The extract increases bladder elasticity and lowers the plasma concentrations of hormones associated with BPH.

Pygeum extract is prescribed in six- to eight-week cycles, with a one-week break in between.

Saw Palmetto Berry (*Serenoa repens*)

A small palm tree native to the southeastern U.S., the saw palmetto produces orange berries that, despite their rancid odor, may be the best therapy for benign prostatic hyperplasia. The berry has a long tradition of medicinal use, for it was employed by Native American healers for genital and urinary disorders. In addition, it enjoys a reputation as an aphrodisiac. Concentrated extracts of saw palmetto berry are the most widely prescribed prostate medications in Germany, France and other European countries, where orthodox physicians routinely use botanical medicines as well as pharmaceutical drugs. Saw palmetto inhibits the conversion of testosterone to dihydrotestosterone, speeds the breakdown and elimination of other hormones implicated in prostate enlargement and reduces both inflammation and the accumulation of fluid.

In a study of 563 patients, those who took saw palmetto extract for three months reported a rate of urine flow twice that of patients who took the prostate drug finasteride (Proscar) for a year. In another study, the 238 patients receiving saw palmetto reported significant relief of overall clinical symptoms within one month. At least seven double-blind, placebo-controlled clinical trials have reported that saw palmetto extracts relieve all major symptoms of BPH. Symptom evaluation and quantitative measurement showed increased urinary flow and a reduction in frequency of urination, residue volume, prostate volume, nighttime urination and difficult or painful urination. No toxicity or significant side effects have been observed.

Health food stores sell saw palmetto berry capsules, tablets, extracts and tinctures. According to a review of saw palmetto literature published in *The Protocol Journal of Botanical Medicine,* hexane extracts of the fruit may have benefits beyond those found in alcohol tinctures. However, none of the clinical trials involving humans have been conducted with alcohol tinctures, so the significance of this difference remains untested. Many American men have reported excellent results from saw palmetto berry capsules and tinctures. Remember that tincture labels give extremely small dosage recommendations; for best results, start with a dropperful once or twice a day and work up to a teaspoon 2 or 3 times daily. For capsules, follow label directions. If no improvement occurs after one month, double the dosage or try another brand.

Because tinctures can be expensive, consider making your own with dried saw palmetto berries purchased from a reputable herb company. To make a potent medicinal tincture, cover 1 cup dried berries with enough 80-proof rum or vodka, or alcohol combined with vegetable glycerine, to fill a quart jar. Seal tightly, leave in a warm place and shake the jar every few days for a month, replenishing the liquid as it is absorbed. At the end of the month, place 1 cup dried berries in another quart jar and strain the tincture from the first jar into the second. Add enough alcohol to fill the container, then repeat the tincturing process: let it stand, shaking the jar every few days, for another four weeks. At the end of the second month, you will have a 2-1/2 month supply of a high quality, medicinal-strength tincture. Take 1 teaspoon twice a day. Use the same procedure to make hawthorn berry tincture for the heart.

As demand for saw palmetto grows, so does concern about its availability. There are no saw palmetto farms or plantations, and demand is beginning to exceed supply. Harvesting saw palmetto berries is itself a risky business, for rattlesnake bites have killed several collectors. We can expect prices to rise as more of the world's men discover the virtues of this highly effective herb—and, as has happened with ginseng and other expensive herbs, we can expect to see product adulteration and other misrepresentations. Be sure to purchase your saw palmetto berries from reputable dealers.

HERBS FOR STRESS AND INSOMNIA

If there is an epidemic among American men, it is probably stress. A little stress may make life more interesting, but constant unresolved stress has been linked to every illness from heart disease to rheumatoid arthritis, cancer, asthma, diverticulitis and other digestive disorders, impotence and depression.

Stress takes a nutritional toll, and no herbs can compensate for the deficiencies of vitamins, minerals, amino acids and other nutrients common to those in high-pressure jobs who live on fast food, coffee and cigarettes. Trace mineral supplements, vitamins and an improved diet do much to reduce the debilitating effects of stress. So do all of the following herbs.

Black Cohosh (*Cimicifuga racemosa*)

Best known as a tonic for the female reproductive system, black cohosh is also found in herbal blends of interest to men, including those for the treatment of insomnia, rheumatism, arthritis, neurological pain and sciatica. A useful antispasmodic, black cohosh helps treat all nervous conditions, cramps and pains. This herb should be taken in small doses because large quantities can be toxic. It is often combined with other relaxing herbs, which reduces its dosage without interfering with its effectiveness.

Chamomile (*Matricaria chamomilla* or *Anthemis nobilis*)

Chamomile blossoms are a widely used, highly effective, calming herb used to help prevent anxiety, improve sleep, prevent gastrointestinal distress and improve digestion. Usually taken as an infused tea, chamomile is also popular in tinctures. Applied externally, chamomile helps prevent swelling and inflammation; cold wet chamomile tea bags are a traditional therapy for under-eye circles. The herb is widely used in skin care products.

Hops (*Humulus lupulus*)

The same blossoms (strobiles) that flavor beer are a specific for the nervous and digestive systems. Hops eases tension, anxiety, indigestion and headaches, but the herb is not recommended for depression. Traditionally used in the treatment of gonorrhea and painful erections, hops is still considered an important herb for men. Its taste is so bitter that it's usually blended with other herbs in teas and tinctures. Hops capsules are an effective treatment for insomnia.

Kava Kava (*Piper methysticum*)

One nervine with a special affinity for today's men is kava kava, a Polynesian herb with a colorful history that calms the nerves without dulling the mind. Kava kava was traditionally prepared not as a tea but as a fermented beverage. With song and ceremony, young girls with strong teeth chewed kava roots until they were reduced to a soft pulp, which they spat into wooden bowls, mixed with coconut milk and kneaded by hand. After hours of fermentation, the liquid was strained off and the result was a potent narcotic used in tribal ceremonies.

Polynesian tribes no longer chew and ferment their kava kava. Instead, they simply crush the roots, mix them with water or coconut milk and filter the liquid. The resulting beverage has a stimulating, tonic effect without being addictive.

Safety is a concern in any discussion of kava kava, for some herbal references dismiss the plant as potentially habit-forming, deservedly notorious and of unproven safety. However, in a report prepared for the *Townsend Letter for Doctors,* herbalist Kerry Bone reviewed the herb's pharmacology and concluded,

> Kava is a safe stabilizing treatment for anxiety, which at normal therapeutic doses does not dampen alertness or interact with mild alcohol consumption. Unlike the benzodiazepine drugs, there is no risk of tolerance or addiction with kava. Its slight antidepressant activity makes it particularly suitable for the treatment of anxiety associated with minor forms of depression. Kava is one of the few safe skeletal muscle relaxants known in the plant kingdom. This property makes it useful for the treatment of nervous tension and conditions associated with skeletal muscle spasm and tension, such as headaches due to neck tension. Although pharmacological tests indicate that kava is not a sedative in the same sense as the antipsychotic and benzodiazepine drugs, it is an excellent hypnotic for the treatment of mild insomnia.

In a double-blind, placebo-controlled study of 58 patients whose anxiety was not caused by psychiatric disorders, kava extract significantly reduced depression and anxiety. Recent German studies demonstrate that kava is a "safe, nonaddictive antianxiety medicine that is as effective as prescription drugs such as Valium."

Long-term use of large quantities of kava causes a distinctive pigmented, dry, scaly skin lesion, which quickly disappears when the herb is discontinued. Adverse effects of kava usage in an Australian aboriginal community resulted from extremely high doses, more than 310 grams (1.2 pounds) per week, and some researchers speculate that large quantities of alcohol may have contributed to kava's toxicity.

The recommended dosage, 1 to 3 grams per day of the powdered dry root in capsules or 1 to 1-1/2 tsp. of kava tincture per day, has caused no adverse side effects in trials lasting up to eight weeks of continuous use.

Passionflower or **Maypop** (*Passiflora incarnata*)

The dried leaves of this climbing vine have a sedative, relaxing, antispasmodic influence that makes it an herb of choice for insomnia, nerve pain such as neuralgia or shingles, asthma or muscle spasms and seizures. Passionflower relaxes without causing drowsiness. It is often combined with valerian, hops, chamomile and other relaxing herbs in teas, tinctures, capsules and tablets.

Skullcap (*Scutellaria lateriflora*)

One of the safest and most effective sedative herbs, skullcap relaxes the nerves without causing drowsiness or interfering with physical coordination. It is used to treat nerve-related disorders such as epilepsy, neuralgia, alcohol withdrawal symptoms, insomnia, stress and anxiety.

Skullcap is often combined with chamomile, hops, passionflower and other relaxing nervines. It is an important ingredient in some stop-smoking programs, for it helps relieve nicotine cravings.

Valerian Root (*Valeriana officinalis*)

The root and rhizome of valerian, also known as garden heliotrope, are beyond aromatic—their odor is so strong that it fills the room, and there's no disguising it. Some call the fragrance earthy, others say valerian smells like old socks and a few dislike the odor so much they refuse to take it.

But for those who can swallow valerian tinctures, tablets, capsules or tea, the rewards are the reduction of high blood pressure, relaxation under stress, relief from pain and a good night's sleep. Valerian does not interfere with a person's ability to drive or operate machinery; in fact, it has been shown to increase efficiency.

Not everyone finds valerian relaxing, however. An estimated 5 to 7 percent of those who try it react with increased agitation and hyperactivity, the exact opposite of what most users experience. If you have never taken valerian, start with half the recommended dosage and monitor your response. If your pulse accelerates or if you feel at all uncomfortable or anxious, discontinue use.

Valerian is one root that should not be boiled as a decoction. Its volatile oils are so fragile, the root should be brewed as an infusion. Pour 2 cups boiling water over 2 tsp. or 1 Tbsp. dried herb, cover, let stand 10 to 15 minutes, strain and serve.

Tonic Herbs

A tonic is an herb that restores and strengthens the entire body, restoring normal tone, stimulating digestion, improving the immune system, and increasing energy, vigor and strength. Some tonic herbs are also "alteratives" or blood cleansers; others are "adaptogens" or herbs that bring the body back into balance by raising or lowering blood pressure, speeding or slowing the pulse and adjusting other systems as needed.

Burdock Root (*Arctium lappa*)

Called gobo in Japan, where it is a common vegetable sold in markets and sushi bars, burdock root is a blood-cleansing herb and general tonic that promotes kidney function and helps clear the blood of harmful acids. In France, fresh burdock root is used to lower blood sugar and is prescribed for diabetics. Erroneous reports of toxicity in burdock stem from a single instance in which burdock root was contaminated with belladonna, which contains the poisonous compound atropine. The incident was never repeated, but some medical authorities still refer to the atropine content of burdock root.

Burdock root should be brewed as a decoction (simmer 1 Tbsp. dried root in 2 cups water for 10 to 15 minutes), and it is often combined with dandelion root, which has similar properties, and other herbs.

Garlic (*Allium sativum*)

Garlic has been used for thousands and thousands of years—for so long, in fact, that its medicinal and culinary applications are older than our written records. Sanskrit manuscripts show that garlic was used as a remedy 5,000 years ago, and the Chinese have been using garlic for at least 3,000 years. The Codex Ebers, an Egyptian medical papyrus compiled in 1550 B.C., describes garlic as effective in treating a variety of ailments, including worms, tumors and headaches. In other cultures, garlic has been recommended for the treatment of sore throats, toothaches, coughs, dandruff, earaches, infections, hypertension, atherosclerosis, hysteria and diarrhea.

Garlic contains 33 sulfur compounds, 17 amino acids and several minerals, including germanium, calcium, copper, iron, potassium, magnesium, selenium and zinc. In addition, it contains vitamins A, B and C.

In the 1940s the substance allicin was discovered. It is a chemically unstable, colorless liquid that provides garlic's pungent odor. For several years, allicin was believed to be the most active ingredient in garlic, accounting for its therapeutic benefits. That claim is still made by the makers of garlic supplements. However, more recent research has shown that garlic contains several ingredients that help improve health. Allicin, because it is so unstable, is difficult to preserve in any manufactured supplement, and the benefits of a high allicin supplement may not be superior to those of other brands. Of course, fresh garlic is an excellent source of not only allicin but all of garlic's compounds.

An impressive body of research documents the many benefits of the pungent clove, especially with regard to heart disease and the circulatory system. In addition to those benefits, garlic has been shown to help prevent cancer; it apparently has an antitumor effect. Garlic is also antiviral, antifungal, antiparasitic, antiprotozoan and antibacterial. Research conducted 50 years ago showed that both garlic juice and allicin inhibit the growth of *staphylococcus, streptococcus, brucella, salmonella,* mycobacteria and other gram-positive and gram-negative bacteria. This makes it of interest to researchers dealing with AIDS, diarrhea, candidiasis, genital herpes, ear infections and a variety of other illnesses.

Many herbalists recommend taking 1 to 3 cloves of garlic daily, raw or cooked. Raw garlic contains more antimicrobial properties, but cooked garlic has a long history of health benefits, and garlic bread, roasted garlic, garlic-laden pesto and slowly simmered garlic-curry sauces are all said to improve the health. To reduce the social side effects of heavy garlic consumption, look for breath products that work from the inside out, such as Breath Assure, which are guaranteed to keep breath fresh no matter what you eat. Or, if internal breath aids aren't available, eat as much chlorophyll as you can in the form of green vegetables such as parsley.

Odorless garlic supplements have become very popular and are sold in supermarkets, pharmacies, health food shops and mail order catalogs. By far the most scientific research has investigated Kyolic brand, an aged extract of extremely pungent garlic grown in Japan. However, studies conducted in Germany and other countries show that other types provide health benefits as well. Capsule or tablet size and strength vary by brand; follow package directions. When fighting an acute infection, such as a cold or the flu, take up to three or four times the recommended dose for several days.

Although garlic supplements have no adverse side effects, and fresh garlic's only problems are its odor and, in large quantities, some digestive disturbance, garlic does have one significant danger. Health officials warn that homemade garlic oil, consisting of olive oil and garlic, can harbor botulism. Commercial garlic-and-oil preparations are now required to contain lemon juice, vinegar or other acidifying ingredients or to be processed at high temperatures to prevent the growth of botulism bacteria. The traditional recipe of letting garlic and olive oil stand in sunlight for several days is considered unsafe for internal consumption. In addition, using fresh, full strength garlic on the skin can burn or blister. Garlic diluted in oil or strong garlic tea is a better choice.

In the past 50 years, garlic research has generated over 2,000 scientific papers and a wealth of evidence supporting traditional claims. A clove of garlic may offer more protection than the apple a day that keeps the doctor away.

Ginseng (*Panax ginseng, P. quinquefolius, Eleutherococcus senticosus*)

Ginseng, an unassuming leafy plant that's both hard to grow and expensive, is the world's most researched medicinal herb, and it is practically synonymous with men's health, especially for those over 40. Since the 17th century it has been the subject of over 3,000 books and papers, but the result of this international investigation has done little to reduce the controversy surrounding ginseng.

There are eight ginseng species, but only three are widely used: *Panax ginseng,* also called Korean ginseng, *Panax quinquefolius,* or American ginseng and *Eleutherococcus senticosus,* or Siberian ginseng. Research shows their effects are similar, though experts disagree on their potency and application. All of the ginseng species are adaptogens, a classification of herb with broad health benefits similar to a tonic. Adaptogens help boost the immune system, improve stamina and endurance, correct imbalances and reduce stress. Korean and American ginseng have been used for centuries; Siberian ginseng is a modern discovery with no tradition of folk use before being tested by Russian scientists.

Ginseng has been shown to prevent the depletion of adrenal hormones, which fight stress; improve memory; increase the body's production of antibodies and chemicals that fight viruses; reduce cholesterol while increasing high-density lipoproteins (HDLs); reduce blood clotting, thus reducing the risk of heart attack; reduce blood sugar levels, thus helping control diabetes; reduce cell damage from radiation; prevent liver damage; counteract fatigue and improve the health of the elderly. In addition, ginseng is an antioxidant, which helps prevent cumulative cell damage leading to cancer. Its most popular reputation is as a tonic for the male reproductive system, and some say it has aphrodisiac powers. Although there is no human study to substantiate this last claim, experiments with laboratory mice showed increased mating activity in the ginseng-using group.

But for every study proving the herb's efficacy, another concludes it has no effect at all. Critics have always suspected researcher bias, for or against, and poor project design for contradictory findings, but a more likely cause is the adulteration of ginseng with other herbs and inefficient preparation techniques. Because ginseng is so expensive, adulteration has always been a problem. A 1978 study of 54 commercial ginseng products showed that 60 percent contained too little of the herb to have any biological effect. In fact, 25 percent contained no ginseng at all. Another adulterant is ginseng itself—that is, the use of immature roots. The active constituents of ginseng increase with the plant's age, and roots should be at least six years old before harvest. Last, most of the active constituents are in the root bark, not the pulp. Researchers who used ginseng root pulp found the herb ineffective.

Is ginseng safe? The literature indicates that ginseng should not be used by anyone suffering from asthma, emphysema, fever, irregular heartbeat, high blood pressure or anxiety disorders. But individual responses vary, and some of these conditions, such as irregular heartbeat and high blood pressure, have in many cases been corrected by ginseng. As noted, information about this herb is often contradictory.

More publicized is "Ginseng Abuse Syndrome," coined in 1979 by the *Journal of the American Medical Association.* An informal poll was taken of 133 psychiatric patients who were also ginseng users, some of whom consumed up to 15 grams of ginseng daily (over twice the highest recommended dose), inhaled or injected the herb (bizarre applications by any standards) or took it with large amounts of coffee. It was reported that most of these users experienced symptoms ranging from morning diarrhea to nervousness, insomnia and elevated blood pressure. All of these side effects are associated with caffeine and the inaccurately-named laxative plant "desert ginseng," which several patients took by mistake (it is not a ginseng species). The report, which has been criticized for its unjustified conclusions, continues to be quoted in medical journals and the press. While any herb can be dangerous if overused, there is no scientific support for Ginseng Abuse Syndrome.

Safety considerations aside, ginseng is not a "magic bullet." It acts so slowly that its effects may not be noticed for weeks or months.

Ginseng can be chewed, steamed, powdered, made into a tincture, used in cooking (the Chinese consider it a pungent root vegetable and add small amounts to soups or stews) or simmered as a tea. Ginseng tea has a slightly bitter taste, but those who drink unsweetened coffee or tea usually find it pleasant. Like most roots, ginseng must be simmered for 10-15 minutes in a covered pan; only powdered ginseng makes an instant tea. My favorite method of ginseng tea preparation is with a ginseng cooker.

The Chinese ginseng cooker is a ceramic pot, rather like a teapot without a handle or spout. It has a flat inner lid and a domed outer lid. The cooker works like a double boiler. Fill it with water, add a piece of ginseng root, put the covers in place and stand the cooker in a pan of boiling water. Reduce the heat and simmer for several hours. If the pan is large enough, cover it with its own lid; this will reduce evaporation. Otherwise, check the water level every hour and add water as necessary to prevent the pan from drying out. A glass jar on a small rack makes an effective ginseng cooker, too.

The water extract produced by the ginseng cooker can be refrigerated and diluted. You can use a full ounce of root in a pint of water, then dilute the resulting tea with three to five times as much water for a daily cup. In this way, a single use of the cooker keeps you supplied with tea for a week and keeps fuel and ginseng costs down without sacrificing quality.

The root can be used once or twice more, although the resulting tea will be weaker. You can combine an old piece with a new one to maintain the brew's strength without wasting any ginseng. Ginseng roots are white (dried) or red (steamed and dried). The red root is more expensive and is said to be more effective. Tea from white root turns brown as it brews, while tea made from red root remains clear. The more bitter the taste, the stronger the brew.

Most of the ginseng sold in Asia today comes from the United States and most of America's ginseng is grown in Wisconsin. Hsu's Ginseng Enterprises in Wausau, Wisconsin, one of the world's largest ginseng producers, recommends that dried ginseng root be steamed or warmed at low heat for five to ten minutes to make it easier to slice, although you can often break a piece without much trouble. The root can be chewed, brewed into tea or made into a concentrated tincture by covering one or more roots with vodka and shaking the jar every day for a month.

It is difficult to say how much ginseng to take because preparations vary as much as the people taking them. In general, the smaller the person, the smaller the dose. The typical recommendation for a 150-pound adult is 5 to 7 grams (1/5 to 1/4 ounce by weight) of high quality root daily, which is roughly equivalent to a one half teaspoon of tincture twice a day or 1 to 2 cups of tea, depending on strength.

Ginseng experts recommend that you take ginseng on an empty stomach or between meals, that the tea be comfortably warm or hot and never served cold and that you drink it in sips during the day rather than all at once. Chinese herbalists recommend that you wait at least three hours after taking ginseng before eating citrus fruits, tomatoes and other foods high in vitamin C. If possible, avoid sweetening your tea. If you can't drink ginseng straight, use honey or raw sugar in small quantities and try to use a little less each time, or sweeten the tea with the herb stevia. Ginseng may be taken in small daily doses, every other day or every week, for several weeks or months at a time.

Obviously, if you experience any discomfort or adverse side effects, discontinue use.

HERBS FOR THE BLADDER, KIDNEYS AND URINARY TRACT

Bladder and kidney health concerns go hand in hand with the older man's prostate problems. All of the prostate-friendly herbs are used in teas and tinctures that support the urinary tract, and the following herbs are considered specifics for this system. You will find them combined with each other and with saw palmetto berry, damiana and other herbs in many formulas.

Buchu (*Agothosma betulina, Barosma betulina*)

An effective diuretic, buchu is one of the best urinary tonics. In large doses, it has a pronounced laxative effect.

Buchu is mostly used to treat such urinary problems as bladder infections, fluid retention and gravel. The American herbalist Michael Tierra recommends treating painful urination with a cold medicinal-strength tea. When taken warm or hot, buchu tea produces perspiration, reduces prostate swelling and soothes irritation of the urethra. Brew as an infusion; do not boil the leaves.

Cranberry

The festive red cranberry, one of the most astringent fruits known, is an effective urinary tract cleanser. Unsweetened cranberry juice and cranberry concentrates are often recommended for kidney and bladder infections, for antiseptic compounds in the berry prevent infectious bacteria from adhering to bladder, kidney and urinary tract walls and tissue. Cranberries are a support therapy for prostate problems.

Cornsilk (*Zea mays*)

The next time you shuck an ear of corn, especially if it's organically grown, consider saving the silk. Those golden threads are a highly regarded urinary tonic, useful in the treatment of urinary tract infections and prostatitis. Often combined with other herbs, cornsilk is used as a tea, in capsules and in tinctures.

Goldenrod (*Solidago viga-aurea*)

The flowers of European goldenrod are gathered in late summer for the treatment of intestinal, kidney and bladder complaints. A kidney stimulant, goldenrod increases the elimination of fluid. For this reason, it is often combined with other herbs in blends for the prostate and urinary tract.

Gravel Root or **Joe Pye Weed** (*Eupatorium purpurea*)

Also called queen of the meadow, the roots of this enormous, purple-blossomed roadside plant have diuretic, astringent and tonic properties. Considered a specific for the bladder and urinary tract, gravel root is named for its ability to rid the body of small stones. A diuretic, gravel root increases the flow of urine. Often combined with uva ursi and marshmallow root, gravel root is an ingredient in urinary tonic blends and prostate formulas.

Juniper Berries (*Juniperus communis*)

The fragrant blue berries of the juniper bush are diuretic, antiseptic and carminative, making them a natural tonic for the kidney, bladder and urinary tract. Juniper berries are often added in small amounts to herbal blends. Because large quantities and frequent consumption may irritate the kidneys, juniper berries should be consumed with caution. Most authorities recommend that this herb not be taken for more than six weeks without a month-long interruption.

The famous European herbalist Father Kneipp started with 2 berries in tea per day, adding 1 or 2 berries daily until reaching 15 berries on the 10th day, then reducing the dosage on the same schedule. This therapy cleanses the kidneys, liver, blood, stomach and urinary tract, and it can be helpful to those with gout for it stimulates the excretion of uric acid through the urine.

Pipsissewa or **Prince's Pine** (*Chimaphila spp.*)

Often found in diuretic, urinary tract and prostate formulas, pipsissewa is both gentle and effective, relieving irritation, improving circulation and healing congestion.

Pipsissewa combines well with dandelion and other herbs.

Uva Ursi or **Bearberry** (*Arctostaphylos uva-ursi*)

This highly astringent leaf is often called a diuretic, but it does little to increase the flow of urine. Instead, it is one of the most effective urinary antiseptics known. Inflammation and infection of the bladder, kidneys and urethra respond well to uva ursi, which is blended with buchu, marshmallow and corn silk to treat kidney stones or gravel, cystitis and pyelitis, a kidney infection in men resulting from stagnant urine blocked by an enlarged prostate or kidney stones.

According to Rudolf Weiss, author of the German textbook *Herbal Medicine,* uva ursi leaves contain 10 percent arbutin, its most important active principle, and 15 percent tannin. Given over extended periods, tannins irritate the stomach, so uva ursi is not recommended for long-term use. Unlike most leaves, uva ursi does not release its active ingredient when combined with boiling water in an infusion. Instead, it should be simmered as a decoction for half an hour. Weiss recommends adding one tablespoon herb to two cups water, then boiling the tea down to one cup in an open pan. Dilute with water or other teas and drink throughout the day, or take ½ teaspoon tincture three times daily in juice, tea or water.

Herbs to Help You Stop Smoking

If you have a respiratory illness, smoking will make it worse. If you live with a smoker, secondhand smoke will do the same. People still argue about the links between smoking and heart disease, but the links between smoking and emphysema, asthma, lung cancer and other respiratory problems are well-documented. Chewing tobacco, which has gained in popularity in recent years, has its own adverse side effects, including cancers of the mouth and throat.

The herbs most helpful to smokers who are trying to quit include the relaxing sedative herbs valerian, chamomile, skullcap, oatgrass and passionflower. The most effective way to use these herbs in a stop-smoking program, when nerves tend to frazzle, is as tinctures (alcohol and/or vegetable glycerine extracts) rather than teas or capsules.

Some herbalists have designed elaborate schedules of dosages (one is described in my book *Herbs to Help You Breathe Freely*), but experimentation is often the best approach. Taken in ¼ to ½ tsp. doses every hour or two throughout the day, none of these tinctures will interfere with alertness or the ability to drive or operate machinery.

It's a good idea to try these tinctures separately after studying their descriptions. Judge their individual effects and test them again as combinations. You can take them on a regular schedule or squirt a dropperful under your tongue whenever you feel the craving for a cigarette or whenever you need to relax. And even though tinctures are more concentrated and faster acting, you can certainly brew these herbs as teas and drink them throughout the day. In fact, you'll find them in "stop smoking" tea blends in the health food store.

If you chew tobacco and would like to stop, your health food store may carry a ginseng "chew" designed for just this purpose. Or simply chew on a dried ginseng root.

Aromatherapy for Men

Aromatherapy is the therapeutic use of fragrances to positively influence our moods and health. Any scent, such as the spicy fragrance of a hot apple pie, can influence both mind and body. In aromatherapy the essential oils distilled from the blossoms, leaves and roots of fragrant plants are used to enhance well-being. Not fats themselves, the oils combine well with vegetable oils, waxes and fats. Alcohol dissolves them partially. They do not dissolve in water.

Essential oils are expensive for good reason: it takes several pounds of fresh plant material to produce even a fraction of an ounce of essential oil. Fortunately, a little goes a long way. Because of their expense, quality is always a concern. Here is a simple test to be sure an essential oil has not been diluted with a carrier oil. Place a drop of the oil on absorbent paper and let it dry. Does it leave an oily stain? If it doesn't, you have a true essential oil.

The essential oils of seemingly identical plants can vary noticeably. For example, two lavender oils may differ because they were made from different species of lavender or because the plants were grown in different regions. When you find an oil you enjoy, buy more than one brand for comparison.

Essential oils are so concentrated that they are rarely used full strength. They can be diluted in carrier oils, such as almond oil, for use as massage oils or added to boiling water to create fragrant steam for air freshening, complexion care or to clear sinus congestion. To make an essential oil water-soluble for use in the bath or as an airspray, insect repellent or skin splash, combine it with enough vodka or other alcohol to dissolve it; then add water. Isopropyl rubbing alcohol is not recommended because of its pronounced medicinal smell, which interferes with natural fragrances.

Lavender, sandalwood and tea tree oils can be applied full strength to most adult skin, but other oils should be diluted first as some essential oils cause burns and blisters. Even well-tolerated oils should be tested by first-time users; if any rash or irritation develops, dilute the oil.

There are many ways to scent a living room or bedroom for relaxation, stress reduction, a good night's sleep, an energy boost in the afternoon or romance. A nebulizer is an electric pump that diffuses essential oils and disperses them into the air in a fine mist. Another air freshener is a candle diffuser, similar to a ceramic potpourri warmer, which heats essential oils combined with water and releases their fragrance slowly. Even a light bulb can be an aromatherapy appliance: place a drop of essential oil on a cold bulb, turn it on and slowly the bulb's heat will release the scent. Ceramic and fiber rings that fit over light bulbs are often sold at aromatherapy counters.

Facial steam treatment. Pour boiling water into a large bowl, add 8 to 10 drops essential oil and, with a large towel, cover your head and the bowl so you're inside a steamy tent. Keep your face several inches above the bowl at all times; the steam is hot enough to burn if you get too close. Try to stay inside the tent for five minutes, coming out for air when necessary. This procedure softens the beard, helps prevent ingrown hairs and tones the skin. To relieve the sinus congestion of colds or hay fever, add eucalyptus, tea tree or peppermint oil to the boiling water.

Sports injuries. For a massage oil that speeds the healing of strained muscles, sprains or sports injuries, add 40 to 60 drops of essential oil, such as tea tree oil or a blend of eucalyptus, fir, lavender, chamomile, cypress, rosemary or juniper, to 1/2 cup (4 fluid ounces) carrier oil. Carrier oils include olive, almond, jojoba, grapeseed, canola, apricot kernel or any light, natural oil.

Prostate massage oil. Combine 5 drops each of lavender and thyme oils, 10 drops cypress or fir, 10 drops eucalyptus or rosemary and 1 fluid oz. (2 Tbsp.) carrier oil. Gently massage over the prostate region and lower back every night before bed.

Foot odor. Use full-strength lavender, sandalwood or tea tree oil on the soles of the feet and work it in well between and around the toes. This treatment works best after a hot footbath to which you have added 1/2 cup salt and several drops of eucalyptus oil.

Jock itch, athlete's foot, toenail fungus. Prepare a dilute solution of tea tree oil by mixing 2 Tbsp. (1 oz.) tea tree oil with sufficient vodka or grain alcohol to dissolve it completely, leaving no oil floating on the surface. Add enough water to measure 3/4 cup (6 fluid oz.) altogether. The resulting solution is approximately 15 percent tea tree oil. Optional additions: Add 1/2 tsp. liquid grapefruit seed extract, which is another powerful fungicide, and several drops of lavender, rosemary, thyme or sage oils. At least twice a day, saturate the affected area with this solution and air dry or use a hair dryer set on low heat. Dust with an antiseptic powder or tea tree oil powder to keep the area dry. Avoid synthetic fabrics and wear cotton or silk socks and underwear. With foot problems, go barefoot as often as possible. Fungal infections thrive in dark, moist conditions; fabrics that breathe and exposure to air and light help prevent a recurrence.

Hemorrhoids or anal itching. Apply a blend of equal parts geranium, lavender and peppermint oils mixed with a small amount of water or use a dilute solution of tea tree oil.

Balanitis, an inflammation of the foreskin not caused by venereal disease. Wash the area twice daily with a gentle soap, rinse well and towel dry. Add 5 drops tea tree oil and lavender or chamomile oil to 1 tsp. salt; mix well, dissolve in 1 cup warm water and bathe the affected area thoroughly. Towel dry. Do not apply full-strength tea tree oil to mucous membranes.

Baldness. Although there is no well-documented cure for baldness, the essential oils of basil, cedarwood, cinnamon, cypress, geranium, ginger, juniper, lemon, neroli, sage and rosemary are considered hair growth stimulators, as is the herb stinging nettle. If it's possible to restore or stimulate hair growth, these essential oils will do so within four to six months of daily use. Combine all or most of the above oils in equal (or approximately equal) quantities.

Every night, add 2 or 3 drops of the essential oil blend to 1/2 tsp. water and massage it vigorously into the scalp, concentrating on areas of hair loss. If you have one, use an electric massager with a hair and scalp attachment. If not, stretch the skin in as many directions as possible. Increase circulation to the scalp by bending over or resting on a slant board as often as possible.

In the morning, shampoo and rinse well. Increase circulation to the scalp by applying a cold washcloth, then a hot one, alternating every 15 or 20 seconds for about two minutes. If your hair is dark, massage the scalp with nettle tea.

Every two weeks, combine several drops of the essential oil blend with enough jojoba or olive oil to cover the entire scalp. Work in well, then cover the head with a towel. Leave undisturbed for as long as possible, preferably overnight. Wash hair and scalp thoroughly in the morning.

In addition, take circulatory herbs such as gotu kola, ginkgo and cayenne. Wild yam (page 29) has been reported to correct some cases of male pattern baldness.

After-shave lotion. Prepare a tincture of rum and bay leaf by filling a pint jar with aromatic bay leaves and cover the leaves with rum. Leave in a warm place and shake the jar daily for a month. Combine 1 Tbsp. tincture with several drops of any masculine, woody or spicy oils, such as basil, cedarwood, cinnamon, clove, cypress, geranium, ginger, juniper, lemon, neroli, nutmeg, sage, rosemary and/or tea tree oils in any combination. If you don't like the result, discard it and start over, keeping track of your oils and proportions, but remember that working with full-strength oils can dull your sense of smell. Before applying to the skin, go for a walk in fresh air and test again. Remember to add only a few drops of oil; very strong fragrances can repel the very people you want to attract. Aim for something subtle and understated. Before using, dilute the tincture-oil blend with an equal quantity of water. When you have created an after-shave lotion that's to your liking, make a larger quantity using the same essential oils.

Insect repellent. Use the same rum and bay leaf tincture to prepare an effective insect repellent. Citronella, bay leaf, lemon, clove, peppermint, myrrh, pennyroyal, eucalyptus, rosemary and tea tree oils repel flies, mosquitoes, ants and fleas. According to herbalists who experiment with live ticks, the most effective tick repellent is rose geranium.

When preparing an insect repellent, you want something substantially stronger than an after-shave lotion, so double or triple the amount of essential oil. Experiment until you find a combination that keeps the bugs away and that you don't mind wearing. Store the repellent in a spray bottle for easy application. After several months of use, essential oils in the repellent may cause the spray bottle's rubber seals to deteriorate and need replacing.

Aromatherapy books, brochures, charts and guidelines are widely published, and most feature essential oils for men. Warm, invigorating fragrances help reduce emotional stress, eliminate fatigue and inspire confidence; these include eucalyptus, cinnamon, pine, rosemary, geranium and bergamot, all of which are useful in cases of sinus congestion, low energy or poor circulation. Soothing herbs help balance energy, refresh the mind and body and strengthen the system; lavender, lemon, sage and lime belong in this category. Chamomile is known for its calming influence and is recommended for the treatment of depression. Sandalwood is deeply relaxing. Lavender helps provide a good night's sleep. Basil, peppermint and juniper are said to aid the memory. Thyme and sandalwood help relieve headaches. Lavender, ylang ylang, patchouli and sandalwood are also romantic, helping set the mood for an intimate evening. But remember, in the romance department, one person's favorite blend is another's "I'm-outa-here" repellent! I've noticed that many men are entranced by patchouli and ylang ylang, which are traditional aphrodisiacs, but some women dislike them intensely. Spend an evening testing scents to determine a mutually acceptable fragrance.

There are over a hundred widely available essential oils. At least one or two of them belong in your life.

Bibliography

Batchelder, H.J., *et al.* "Therapeutic Approaches to Benign Prostatic Hyperplasia." *The Protocol Journal of Botanical Medicine,* Volume 1, Number 3, Winter 1996.

Bone, Kerry. "Kava, a Safe Herbal Treatment for Anxiety." *Townsend Letter for Doctors,* June 1995.

Brewer, Sarah. *The Complete Book of Men's Health.* New York: Thorsons/Harper Collins, 1995.

Burton Goldberg Group. *Alternative Medicine: The Definitive Guide.* Fife, Wash.: Future Medicine Publishing, Inc., 1994.

Christopher, John. *School of Natural Healing.* Springville, Ut.: Christopher Publications, 1978.

Duke, James A. *Handbook of Medicinal Herbs.* Boca Raton, Fla.: CRC Press, 1985.

Foster, Steven, and Duke, James A. *Peterson Field Guides: Eastern/Central Medicinal Plants.* Boston: Houghton Mifflin, 1990.

Green, James. *The Male Herbal: Health Care for Men and Boys.* Freedom, Calif.: Crossing Press, 1991.

Hancock, Ken. *Feverfew: Your Headache May Be Over.* New Canaan, Conn.: Keats Publishing, Inc., 1986.

Hoffmann, David. *An Elder's Herbal.* Rochester, Vt.: Healing Arts Press, 1993.

Lust, John. *The Herb Book.* New York: Bantam Books, 1974.

McTaggart, Lynne. *Medical Madness: How to Prevent the LeadingCause of Poor Health.* Baltimore: What Doctors Don't Tell You, 1995.

Moore, Michael. *Medicinal Plants of the Pacific West.* Santa Fe: Red Crane Books, 1993.

Mowrey, Daniel B. *Proven Herbal Blends: A Rational Approach to Prevention and Remedy.* New Canaan, Conn.: Keats Publishing, Inc., 1986.

Ornish, Dean. *Dr. Dean Ornish's Program for Reversing Heart Disease.* New York: Ballantine, 1990.

Prevention Guides. *Healing Herbs.* Emmaus, Pa.: Rodale Press, Inc., 1996.

Puotinen, CJ. *Herbal Teas.* New Canaan, Conn.: Keats Publishing, Inc., 1996.

———. *Herbs for Arthritis.* New Canaan, Conn.: Keats Publishing, Inc., 1997.

———. *Herbs for Improved Digestion.* New Canaan, Conn.: Keats Publishing, Inc., 1996.

———. *Herbs to Help You Breathe Freely.* New Canaan, Conn.: Keats Publishing, Inc., 1996.

———. *Herbs for the Heart.* New Canaan, Conn.: Keats Publishing, Inc., 1997.

———. *Nature's Antiseptics: Tea Tree Oil and Grapefruit Seed Extract.* New Canaan, Conn.: Keats Publishing, Inc., 1996.

Quinn, Dick. *Death by Deception.* Minneapolis: R.F. Quinn, 1995.

———. *Left for Dead.* Minneapolis: R.F. Quinn, 1992.

Tierra, Michael. *The Way of Herbs.* New York: Pocket Books, 1983.

Treben, Maria. *Health Through God's Pharmacy.* Steyr, Austria: Wilhelm Ennsthaler, 1980.

Tyler, Varro E. *The Honest Herbal.* New York: Pharmaceutical Products Press, 1993.

Walker, Morton. *Sexual Nutrition.* Garden City Park, N.Y.: Avery Publishing Group, 1994.

Weiss, Rudolf Fritz. *Herbal Medicine.* Translated from the Sixth German Edition of *Lehrbuch der Phytotherapie* by A.R. Meuss. Beaconsfield, England: Beaconsfield Publishers Ltd., 1988.

Wertheimer, Neil, editor. *Total Health for Men.* Emmaus, Pa.: Rodale Press, 1995.

Whitaker, Julian. *The Heart Surgery Trap: Why Most Invasive Procedures Are Unnecessary and How to Avoid Them.* New York: Simon & Schuster, 1992.

Worwood, Valerie Ann. *The Complete Book of Essential Oils and Aromatherapy.* San Rafael, Calif.: New World Library, 1991.

Appendix: Resources

Swedish Bitters

To order Swedish bitters dry herb blend for making your own tincture, send $20 in U.S. funds (1996 price quote) to RiPharm, P.O. Box 23, 4710 Grieskirchen, Austria, or write to verify price and availability. Follow directions on page 47.

Organizations

American Botanical Council, P.O. Box 201660, Austin, TX 78720.

American Herb Association, P.O. Box 1673, Nevada City, CA 95959.

Herb Research Foundation, 1007 Pearl Street, Suite 200, Boulder, CO 80302.

Northeast Herbal Association, P.O. Box 479, Milton, NY 12547.

Magazines

The Herb Companion, 201 East 4th Street, Loveland, CO 80537.

The Herb Quarterly, P.O. Box 689, San Anselmo, CA 94960.

HerbalGram, P.O. Box 201660, Austin, TX 78720.

Dried Herbs and Teas by Mail

Avena Botanicals, P.O. Box 365, West Rockport, ME 04865.

Green Terrestrial, P.O. Box 41, Route 9W, Milton, NY 12547.

The Herb Closet, 104 Main Street, Montpelier, VT 05602.

The Herbfarm, 32804 Issaquah Fall City Road, Fall City, WA 98024.

Island Herbs, Ryan Drum, Waldron Island, WA 98297.

Jean's Greens, 54 McManus Road, Rensselaerville, NY 12147.

Mountain Rose Herbs, P.O. Box 2000, Redway, CA 95560.

Richters, Goodwood, Ontario L0C 1A0, Canada.

Sage Mountain Herb Products, P.O. Box 420, East Barre, VT 05649.

Trinity Herbs, P.O. Box 199, Bodega, CA 94992.

Wild Weeds, P.O. Box 88, Redway, CA 95560.

Live Plants and Seeds

Bountiful Gardens, Ecology Action, 5798 Ridgewood Road, Willits, CA 95490. Special varieties, heirloom seeds.

Fox Hollow Herb & Heirloom Seed Company, P.O. Box 148, McGrann, PA 16236.

Gardens Alive, 5100 Schenley Place, Lawrenceburg, IN 47025. Organic gardening supplies.

Le Jardin du Gourmet, St. Johnsbury Center, VT 05863.

Nichols Garden Nursery, 1190 N. Pacific Highway, Albany, OR 97321.

Richters, Goodwood, Ontario L0C 1A0, Canada. Required reading, excellent source, the catalog is itself an herbal. Highly recommended.

Territorial Seed Company, 20 Palmer Avenue, Cottage Grove, OR 97424.

Vermont Wildflower Farm, P.O. Box 5, Route 7, Charlotte, VT 05445.

Wildseed Farms, Inc., 1101 Campo Rosa Road, P.O. Box 308, Eagle Lake, TX 77434.

Index